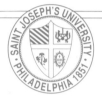

THE PHYSIOLOGY OF NERVE CELLS

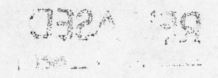

The Physiology of Nerve Cells

BY JOHN CAREW ECCLES

Professor of Physiology

The Australian National University

Canberra

BALTIMORE: The Johns Hopkins Press: 1957

The Physiology of Nerve Cells was first given as a series of
Herter lectures at The Johns Hopkins School of Medicine,
in October, 1955. The lectures were revised and expanded
for this publication by the author, Dr. J. C. Eccles.

Second printing, 1957

© 1957 by The Johns Hopkins Press, Baltimore 18, Md.

Distributed in Great Britain by
the Oxford University Press, London

Printed in U. S. A.

Library of Congress Catalog Card Number 57-7108

FOR MY WIFE, *Irene Frances* *the talking mule*

PREFACE

This book was developed from three lectures that were delivered at The Johns Hopkins University in the fall of 1955. The Johns Hopkins University had honoured me by an invitation to deliver the Twenty-ninth Course of Lectures on the Herter Foundation. The three lectures were entitled:
1. The motor neurone and excitatory synaptic action
2. Inhibitory synaptic action
3. Pathways and transmitter substances in the central nervous system

Each lecture has been amplified considerably and is represented by two chapters of the book. The account given in the lectures has been substantially modified in two fields where more recent investigation has shown that it was erroneous. Otherwise, the changes have consisted merely in the addition of more experimental illustrations of the essential ideas expressed in the lectures.

It is not unreasonable to maintain that nerve cells are more interesting and important than any other cells, being, as they are, the unitary constituents of the nervous system and the functional units responsible for all its multifarious activities, including the amazing performance of the human brain; yet until recently the nerve cell in itself has been understood too little to warrant a monograph. In the last few years, however, the situation has been changed by the application of new and powerful methods, the microtechniques. The greater part of the present monograph is concerned with the intracellular investigation of nerve cells, not only the mere recording of the intracellular potentials evoked in their various reactions, but also the modifications of these potentials that occur during and after the passage of current through an intracellular microelectrode. Such intracellular investigations have been of particular significance in studying the synaptic responses of the individual cell. On the other hand, the extracellular recording of potential fields by microelectrodes has been of great value in elucidating the propagation of impulses over the various components of the individual nerve cells and along pathways formed by two or more cells in synaptic series. Finally, electron-microscopy already has revealed extremely fine structural details which may be correlated with the functional behaviour of the synaptic junctions.

Though these three types of microinvestigations are still at an early stage, so much information has been obtained already that it has seemed opportune to organize it into a monograph. This present account can be regarded as being complementary to a monograph entitled "The Neurophysiological Basis of Mind: The Principles of Neurophysiology," which was written about four years ago, and which gave an account of some of the earliest investigations with intracellular microelectrodes. Already these sections of that monograph have been superseded.

In the earlier book it was recognized that synaptic transmission in the central nervous system was mediated by chemical transmitter substances, but little could be added to this general concept. Even now there has been an identification of only one transmitter at one type of synaptic junction in the central nervous system. Nevertheless, recent experimental work makes it possible to devote a whole chapter to investigations and problems concerning pathways and transmitter substances.

The final chapter is frankly much more speculative, for here the attempt is made to develop ideas that may be of significance in the further investigation and understanding of the nervous system. The title of this chapter is derived from a remarkable book, *Features in the Architecture of Physiological Function,* by Sir Joseph Barcroft, in which the theme was not only that form and function are closely correlatable in living tissues, but also that a form or pattern may be discovered in the functional processes themselves.

There can be no doubt that these concepts will prove particularly fruitful in the central nervous system, where fundamental significance attaches both to the functional and to the structural patterns. The final chapter does not attempt a systematic survey of this whole field. It is merely an attempt to illustrate it by a few examples.

I wish to thank the Committee of The Herter Lectureship, Drs. Lehninger, Harvey, and Rich, of The Johns Hopkins University, for kindly inviting me to give the lectures and for their efforts in making the lectures a success. In addition, I wish to express my gratitude to my numerous friends at Johns Hopkins and in particular to Drs. Bard, Magladery, Kuffler, and Mountcastle. I have been helped greatly in writing this monograph by my neurophysiological colleagues from many countries. The ideas expressed herein were developed not only in discussions with my collaborators here in Canberra, but also with neurophysiologists during the meetings, the colloquia, and the more informal occasions that were so memorable during my overseas visit in 1955. In particular, I would like to thank Drs. Palade, Palay, Bullock, and Hagiwara for kindly allowing me to reproduce illustrations from their unpublished work. I also wish to thank my colleagues P. Fatt, A. Lundberg, J. S. Coombs, D. R. Curtis, A. W. Liley, V. B. Brooks, and Rosamond Eccles, not only for granting me the use of some of the figures, but also for reading and criticizing the manuscript. Finally, I wish to thank Mr. Winsbury, Mr. Daynes, Mr. Chapman, and Mr. Paral, who have helped so much in the design and construction of equipment as well as in the preparation of the illustrations, and Miss R. Burkitt for all her work in the preparation of the manuscript.

ACKNOWLEDGEMENTS

Grateful thanks are due to the following publishers and editors for their generosity in giving permission for the reproduction of figures: *Journal of Physiology; Journal of Neurophysiology; Journal of General Physiology; Quarterly Journal of Experimental Physiology; Nature;* and Charles C. Thomas.

CONTENTS

CONTENTS

CHAPTER I

THE NERVE CELL
AND ITS SURFACE MEMBRANE

A. INTRODUCTION

Cajal (1934, 1954) has told in his characteristically vigorous style the history of the concept that the nervous system is composed of discrete units or nerve cells. The concept was first proposed by His and Forel and then independently by Cajal, while later the name "neurone" was suggested by Waldeyer for the nerve cell and "neurone theory" for the concept of independence of nerve cells. Although all the great neurohistologists of that classical era were ranged for or against the neurone theory, it was pre-eminently the achievement of Cajal to establish that the functional connections between individual nerve cells, or neurones, are effected by close contacts and not by continuity in a syncytial network, as proposed in the rival reticular theory of Gerlach and Golgi. Appropriately Cajal's last great contribution (1934) was devoted to a critical survey of the evidence for and against the neurone theory, which has not been seriously challenged since that time, at least for the vertebrate nervous system.

Sherrington (1897) gave the name "synapse" to these functional connections that are made by close contact between nerve cells. His magnificent contribution to neurology was concerned largely with showing how the reactions of the nervous system could be explained by the integrated behavior of individual nerve cells, each of which functioned as a unit and exerted graded excitatory or inhibitory synaptic actions on other nerve cells (Sherrington, 1906; 1925; 1929; 1931). This functional unity derived from two kinds of reaction. First, the cell integrated the various synaptic excitatory and inhibitory influences, inhibition acting as a quantitative antagonist to excitation. Second, if the unbalanced excitatory influence was sufficiently intense, the cell generated an all-or-nothing impulse which traversed its axon to exert in turn excitatory or inhibitory synaptic influences on other nerve cells, or, if the cell was a motoneurone, to cause contraction of its motor unit. Essentially we can consider the behaviour of the nervous system as being built up from the behaviour patterns of each of its myriad nerve cells, of which the human central nervous system contains more than 10^{10}. This behaviour pattern is defined at any instant by the two possible states of a cell, activation by an impulse or quiescence.

B. THE STRUCTURE AND DIMENSIONS OF NERVE CELLS

Since much of the experimental investigation already performed has dealt with the motor nerve cells (motoneurones) of the mammalian spinal cord, special reference will be made to them. Other nerve cells of widely differing type, however, have now been studied sufficiently to give us assurance that the mammalian motoneurone is providing valid information about nerve cells in general, though in some respects it will be found to exhibit specialized behaviour.

The essential structure of a motoneurone and the synaptic contacts thereon are shown in Figure 1. The diagrammatic representation of the whole motoneurone is derived not only from serial sections, as in the models constructed by Haggar and Barr (1950), but also from remarkable preparations of isolated motoneurones (Chu, 1954). Typically the motoneurone has a cell body or soma approxi-

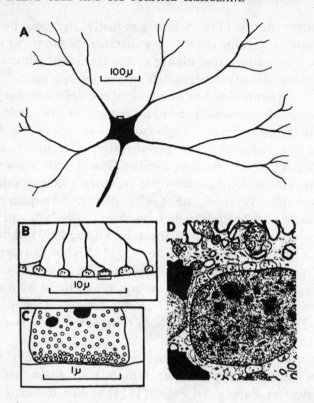

Figure 1 A–D

Drawing of a motoneurone to illustrate general relationships of dendrites and axon to the soma. The small surface area that is outlined is drawn at 20 times higher magnification in *B* to illustrate the relationship of the synaptic knobs to the surface (cf. *D*). The small area outlined in *B* is drawn at 10 times further magnification in *C* to show the width of the synaptic cleft and the thickness of the surface membranes of the synaptic knob and the nerve cell (cf. Figure 1E). Also shown are the synaptic vesicles and mitochondria of the synaptic knob. *D*. Drawing of a low-power photograph obtained with an electronmicroscope showing twelve synaptic knobs in contact with a large dendrite, and also smaller dendrites, on one of which there is a synaptic knob. Note characteristic mitochondria of the knobs (Wyckoff and Young, 1956).

mately 70 μ across, from which radiates a number of branching processes (dendrites) that extend for long distances, as much as 1 mm, before breaking up into fine terminal branches. Also arising from the soma is the axon, or motor nerve fibre, which gradually narrows before assuming a myelin sheath at a distance of some 50 μ to 100 μ. The twenty fold higher magnification of Figure 1B shows the density with which the expanded axonal terminals (synaptic knobs) of other nerve cells encrust the surface of the soma and the basal regions of the dendrites, the distribution being progressively sparser as the dendrites are followed more peripherally (Lorente de Nó, 1938; Barr, 1939; Bodian, 1952). This is well shown in Figure 1D, which is a drawing from an electron microphotograph (Wyckoff and Young, 1956). Synaptic endings have also been described on the axon hillock and the non-medullated segment of the axon (Barr, 1939), though Hoff (1932a) and Lorente de Nó (1938) do not report their presence there with motoneurones. Certainly the density is much less than on the soma, and there is no sign of the specialized synaptic terminals that surround the axonal origin from the Mauthner cells of teleosts (Bodian, 1937; 1940; 1942; 1952).

Finally, in Figure 1C a further ten fold magnification shows schematically the fine structure of a synapse, as described by Palade and Palay (1954) and de Robertis and Bennett (1955), for the synapses on several different types of cells. As revealed in the electron microphotograph (Figure 1E) continuous membranes approximately 50 Å thick cover the synaptic knob and the neuronal soma, there being a cleft approximately 200 Å in width between the two membranes. Within the synaptic knob there are numerous vesicles about 300 Å in diameter, which occasionally are seen opening on the synaptic surface. The mitochondria indicate that there is a high level of metabolic activity in the synaptic knob, which contrasts with the cytoplasm beneath the subsynaptic membrane. Probably, as with the motor nerve endings on muscle (Robertson, 1956; Palade and Palay, 1954), the vesicles of the synaptic knobs may be regarded as containing the chemical substances that are responsible for transmission across the synaptic junctions (cf. Chap. V). It should be noted that,

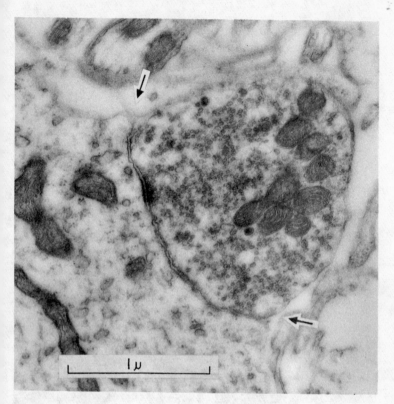

μ 1

Figure 1 E

A very high magnification by electron microscopy to show synaptic knob separated from subsynaptic membrane by a synaptic cleft (marked by arrows) about 200 Å wide. In some areas the vesicles are seen to be concentrated close to the synaptic surface of the knob with the mitochondria lying farther back (Palade and Palay, 1956).

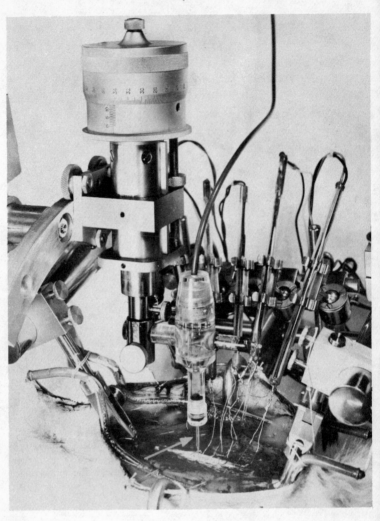

Figure 2

Photograph illustrating some of the apparatus employed in recording intracellularly from nerve cells in cat spinal cord. The rigid attachment of the micromanipulator to the frame that supports the cat is beyond the left of the picture. The spinal cord lies beneath a pool of paraffin oil and the microelectrode (indicated by arrow) is shown protruding downward from the preamplifier and inserted into the spinal cord. The electrodes arranged on the other side of the preparation are employed for such purposes as stimulating ventral roots and leading from the surface of the spinal cord.

in all the following discussions on the responses of neurones, the fine internal structure (cf. Palay and Palade,
1955) has been neglected. The immediate electrical responses and the specific actions of transmitter substances
appear to be surface phenomena, while the deep structures
seem to be concerned with recovery processes, metabolism,
protein manufacture, etc. (cf. Hydén, 1943).

The word synapse, as proposed by Sherrington, may be
applied to the synaptic knob with its chemical mechanism,
the synaptic cleft of 200 Å, and the subsynaptic membrane
with its specific receptive and reactive mechanism. On
analogy with the end-plate membrane of the neuromuscular junction (Kuffler, 1943; Fatt and Katz, 1951;
Castillo and Katz, 1954e; 1955a), it is probable that the
subsynaptic membrane has very different properties from
the remainder of the soma-dendritic membrane, being
specifically affected by the transmitter substance, and
probably being unable to respond to an impulse.

Even in the unstained preparation, the axon hillock and
the non-medullated axon of motoneurones may be distinguished from the soma and dendrites by the absence of
Nissl substance and pigment granules (Chu, 1954); and
as noted above there is much less coverage by synaptic
knobs. Moreover, it will appear later (Chap. II) that on
physiological grounds there is a very remarkable distinction between these two zones of the motoneurone. For
one zone, therefore, it is proposed to make use of the
collective term "initial segment of the axon" or simply
"initial segment," which generally has been applied to the
non-medullated segment of the axon and the axon hillock
from which it arises (cf. Lloyd, 1951a, Lorente de
Nó, 1953).

When inserting a microelectrode, by far the largest
target is presented by the soma and the adjacent large
dendritic branches. In all but a few exceptional experiments we may, therefore, assume that the microelectrode
is implanted therein. It is improbable that with our technique a microelectrode could be implanted satisfactorily in

such tenuous structures as the more distal dendritic branches. Furthermore, on analogy with muscle fibres and giant axons, it is probable that the intracellularly recorded electric potentials arise across the surface membrane of the nerve cell. Investigations on large peripheral nerve cells have the great advantage that the microelectrode actually can be seen within the cell (Tauc, 1954; 1955b; Eyzaguirre and Kuffler, 1955a; Arvanitaki and Chalazonitis, 1955). Such investigations show further that all parts of the cytoplasm are virtually isopotential, which is to be expected, because the cytoplasm is likely to have such a low specific resistance that the currents flowing within the soma would develop only a very small potential. We may, therefore, conclude that the whole surface membrane of the soma has virtually the same potential difference across it, which is that recorded between the intracellular electrode and the indifferent external electrode.

On the contrary the dendrites are so long, relative to their diameter, that changes in the membrane potential of more distal regions would make a negligible contribution to potentials recorded by a microelectrode implanted in the soma. An approximate calculation based on probable values for the specific membrane resistance and for the specific resistance of the cytoplasm reveals that, if a steady change is produced in the membrane potential of a dendrite 5 μ in diameter, only one-half of that potential change will be recorded at a distance of 200 μ along the dendrite from that zone, i.e., the length constant is about 300 μ (Coombs, Eccles, and Fatt, 1955a). Similarly, when currents through the microelectrode are employed to change the ionic composition of the motoneurone, these changes will be restricted largely to the soma and adjacent segments of the dendrites.

Approximate values for the effective volume and surface area of a standard motoneurone may therefore be derived by neglecting the dendrites beyond 300 μ and assuming that the standard motoneurone is a sphere 70 μ in diameter with 6 cylindrical dendrites (cf. Balthasar, 1952) of 5 μ in diameter radiating therefrom for 300 μ, and an axon arising from a conical axon hillock. The volume and surface areas so calculated for a standard motoneurone are approximately $2.5 \times 10^{-7} cm^3$ and $5 \times 10^{-4} cm^2$ respectively if allowance is made for the conical origin of the dendrites from the soma.

Pyramidal cells of the cerebral cortex have a much smaller volume, $2 \times 10^{-8} cm^3$ being the largest soma volume measured by Sholl (1953), and interneurones would be smaller still. The largest sympathetic ganglion cells have a volume of no more than $1 \times 10^{-8} cm^3$. Presumably the relatively small size of interneurones and sympathetic ganglion cells accounts for the difficulty in recording intracellularly from them and for their rapid deterioration under such conditions (R. M. Eccles, 1955). For example, diffusion from the microelectrode would be expected to cause a rapid change in the ionic composition, and there would be an accompanying rapid swelling due to influx of water. On the other hand many nerve cells of invertebrates are quite large. For example, the crustacean stretch receptor cells are at least as large as motoneurones (Figure 32A; Alexandrowicz, 1951; 1952; Florey and Florey, 1955, Eyzaguirre and Kuffler, 1955a), and many ganglion cells of *Aplysia* are very much larger (Tauc, 1954; 1955b; Arvanitaki and Chalazonitis, 1955).

C. TECHNICAL PROCEDURE

Nerve cells of the central nervous system have complex branches, which interlace with the branches of multitudes of other nerve cells from many of which they receive synaptic contacts; hence for physiological investigations it is not feasible to attempt anatomical isolation, as has been done post mortem by Chu (1954). It is possible, however, by intracellular microelectrode techniques (Brock, Coombs, and Eccles, 1952a; 1953; Woodbury and Patton,

1952; Araki, Otani, and Furukawa, 1953; Albe-Fessard and Buser, 1954; Araki and Otani, 1955; Coombs, Eccles and Fatt, 1955a, b, c, and d; Phillips, 1955; 1956a, b; Frank and Fuortes, 1955a, b; 1956a, b) to secure all the advantages that would accrue from anatomical localization, and yet at the same time to have this cell lying virtually unmolested in the central nervous system and being normally supplied with blood. These techniques are so effective that they are the methods of choice for peripheral nerve cells that could be isolated anatomically, e.g., the crustacean stretch receptor cells (Eyzaguirre and Kuffler, 1955a, b) and the ganglion cells of *Aplysia* (Tauc, 1954; 1955b; Arvanitaki and Chalazonitis, 1955).

Essentially the technique requires (cf. Grundfest, 1955) that the surface membrane of the cell be punctured by a very fine glass tube which usually is filled with a salt solution and which acts as an insulated lead from the interior of the cell. The microelectrode, as it is called, has a tip diameter measuring from 0.5μ to 1μ and a resistance usually of from 10 MΩ to 20 MΩ. The other electrical lead is an indifferent lead from a large area of the animal. If mechanical disturbances are reduced by extreme precautions in fixation, the microelectrode is sealed into the surface membrane and the cell may behave normally for several hours. In order to secure these favourable conditions, the animal must be fixed rigidly on a heavy steel frame. A special micromanipulator is used to insert the microelectrode (Figure 2). During the insertion procedure, electrical responses are evoked from the motoneurones so that there is displayed on the cathode ray screen a standing wave which provides information about the proximity of the various groups of motoneurones to the tip of the microelectrode. Penetration of a neurone results in the immediate appearance of the membrane potential and in a drastic change in the signals so recorded, which are inverted and greatly increased in size. The recorded potentials are produced practically entirely by the impaled cell, the reactions of which can thus be studied in isolation from its fellows. In all intracellular records throughout this monograph, potential changes in a positive direction are shown by upward deflections.

Because of its high electrical resistance, the microelectrode must feed into a cathode-follower amplifier, and special precautions must be taken in order to make the capacity of the input to ground as small as possible (cf. Grundfest, 1955). In part, the effect of capacity in producing a poor high-frequency response can be diminished by incorporating a negative capacity device in the amplifier.

The tip diameter of the microelectrode must range within fairly narrow limits. If it is too large, e.g., with a diameter in excess of 1 μ, the surface membrane is likely to be gravely injured by the impalement, and progressive deterioration of the neurone is likely to arise because of the high rate at which ions are diffusing from the electrode into the neurone. For example, if a 3 M-KCl-filled electrode has a resistance of 10 MΩ, it can be calculated that both K^+ and Cl^- ions will diffuse into the neurone at rather less than 0.04 p. mole per second (Coombs, Eccles and Fatt, 1955b), which would cause the Cl^- concentration of the neurone to increase from about 9 mM to 14 mM, if the time constant for diffusional equilibrium of Cl^- ions is 30 sec. (cf. Chapter III). If the tip is too small, e.g., with a resistance over 50 MΩ, the high frequency response of the recording system will be too low, unless a special negative capacity device is introduced, and in addition there is a greatly increased hazard both of electrode blockage by particulate material of the spinal cord and even of the neurone and of spurious values being observed for the resting potential (cf. R. H. Adrian, 1956). If a negative capacity is not introduced, the capacity to ground is usually about 5 $\mu\mu$F, which gives time constants of 50 μsec. and 100 μsec. for input resistances of 10 MΩ and 20 MΩ respectively. Under such conditions the rising phase of the spike potential will be considerably slowed and the summit of the spike potential will be lowered by as much as 20 mV (cf. Brock *et al.*, 1952a).

The ionic composition of a motoneurone can be changed by passing current through a microelectrode that is implanted in it. Because of the much higher ionic concentration in the microelectrode (about 20 times) the current is carried out of the electrode very largely by the passage of the appropriate ion species into the neurone. However, in assessing the change thereby produced in the ionic composition of the neurone, account also has to be taken of the ionic flux that carries the current across the neuronal membrane (Coombs *et al.*, 1955a; 1955b). In particular, most of a current passing outward across the membrane, i.e., a current in the depolarizing direction, is carried by the outward movement of potassium ions, the inward movement of Cl^- ions probably accounting for only about 25 per cent, but this proportion would be increased by potassium depletion (cf. Chapter III). Thus, when a current is passed into the neurone from a microelectrode filled with a sodium salt, sodium ions will be injected into the neurone and will replace the potassium ions that carry the current outward across the surface membrane. It is possible in this way to produce large changes in the ionic composition, for a current of 5×10^{-8}A requires a net ionic movement of 30 p. equiv. per minute. When attempting to estimate the changes so produced in the motoneurone, allowances have to be made for the restitutive changes which will be operating during the injection both by diffusional processes (for Cl^- ions in particular, see Chapter III) and by the operation of the sodium-potassium pump (Fig. 8). When in Figure 26A a current of 4×10^{-8}A was passed into the neurone for 120 sec. from a microelectrode filled with Na_2SO_4 (1.2 equiv. per litre), there would thus be approximate gains of 25 p. equiv. of Na^+ ions and 5 p. equiv. of Cl^- ions and a loss of 20 p. equiv. of K^+ ions. These are relatively large changes, because, on the basis of a volume of 2.5×10^{-7}cm^3 and a concentration of 150 mM, the total K^+ ion content of a motoneurone would be about 35 p. equiv. (Coombs *et al.*, 1955a).

A current in the opposite direction would be passing in through the membrane and thence into the microelectrode, i.e., it would tend to hyperpolarize the membrane. It would flow into the microelectrode largely by movement of anions from it into the neurone, while it would be carried inward across the surface membrane mainly by the inward passage of K^+ ions and the outward passage of Cl^- ions, though inward Na^+ ionic movement would also contribute. In attempting to estimate the ionic changes produced by the passage of these currents, an important consideration is that the net effect is an increase in neutral salt within the cell, which osmotically causes a net influx of water across the membrane.

By means of a double-barrelled microelectrode (Figure 3) it has been possible to subject the neurone to the flow of a steady current which is applied through one barrel in either direction and at the same time to record the potential changes through the other barrel. The application of this technique is described in connection with the measurements of membrane resistance and the electric time constant of the membrane, and with the determination of the equilibrium potentials for the various responses in Chapters II and III.

D. THE ELECTRICAL CONSTANTS OF THE RESTING SURFACE MEMBRANE

1. The Membrane Potential

The membrane potential of the soma has been directly measured as the change in potential observed when the microelectrode penetrates the surface membrane, or is withdrawn across it. Often the potential builds up for several minutes, it being assumed that meanwhile the membrane is sealing around the electrode and preventing short-circuiting currents from flowing from the outside to

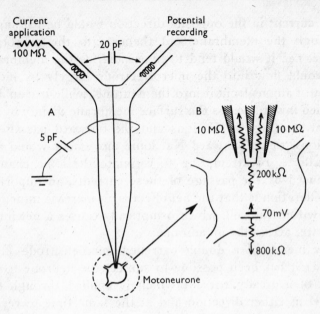

Figure 3

A. Double-barrelled microelectrode and its immediate connexions. Typical values are given for the several electrical characteristics which are significant in the use of the electrode. *B*. Enlarged view of the microelectrode tip in the motoneurone. The motoneurone properties represented are the potential and resistance (ignoring the reactance) between the inside and outside of the inactive cell. For diagrammatic purposes the microelectrode tip is shown greatly magnified relative to the motoneurone. (Coombs, Eccles, and Fatt, 1955a).

the interior of the cell. When values derived from those motoneurones showing grave injury or deterioration are rejected, the membrane potential of motoneurones approximates −70 mV (internal potential relative to the external indifferent electrode), the usual range being from −60 mV to −80 mV (Brock *et al.*, 1952a; Woodbury and Patton, 1952; Coombs *et al.*, 1955a; Frank and Fuortes, 1955b). With pyramidal cells of the cerebral cortex, lower values of about −60 mV were observed by Phillips (1955; 1956a, b), but in part at least this lower value is caused by the background synaptic bombardment. Mammalian sympathetic ganglion-cells likewise have a membrane potential of about −70 mV (R. M. Eccles, 1955). With amphibian motoneurones the membrane potential has usually been from −40 mV to −60 mV (Alanis and Matthews, 1952; Araki *et al.*, 1953; Araki and Otani, 1955). Membrane potentials ranging from −35 mV to −60 mV (mean, −50 mV) have been recorded for the neurones of the electric lobe of the *Torpedo* (Albe-Fessard and Buser, 1954) and from −30 mV to −60 mV for the ganglion cells of *Aplysia* (Tauc, 1954; 1955b; Arvanitaki and Chalazonitis, 1955). Probably the lower values are attributable to cellular injury. With crustacean stretch receptor cells the membrane potential is of the same order as with mammalian motoneurones, −70 mV to −80 mV (Eyzaguirre and Kuffler, 1955a). It is of particular interest that the membrane potential for the axon was found to be identical to that for the soma of the same cell (Eyzaguirre and Kuffler, 1955b). With motoneurones there is also evidence that the same membrane potential obtains for the soma and axon (Coombs *et al.*, 1955a), but less significance attaches to these observations, since they were always made on different motoneurones.

When the ionic composition of a motoneurone is altered by electrophoretic injection of ions (Coombs *et al.*, 1955a, b), there are often considerable changes in the membrane potential. For example, depletion of intracellular potassium is always accompanied by a fall, which may be as large as 30 mV. If the potassium is replaced by sodium, the membrane potential recovers to its initial value within several minutes, and then usually passes over to a prolonged phase of hyperpolarization (filled circles, Figure 44D). Injection of diffusible anions such as Cl⁻ ions also causes a temporary depression of membrane potential, usually by no more than 10 mV, and recovery occurs within two or three minutes.

2. The Membrane Resistance

By employing a double-barrelled microelectrode, it is possible to pass an electric current from one barrel to the indifferent grounded electrode, and to measure the potential change so produced between the other barrel and the indifferent electrode. For the first few milliseconds the recorded potential is attributable mostly to the flow of capacitive currents, but thereafter a virtually steady potential is recorded (Coombs *et al.*, 1955a). In a uniformly conducting medium this steady potential is attributable to the voltage drop in the resistance which is common to the circuits from the orifice of each barrel to the indifferent electrode, and which can be called the coupling resistance between the two barrels. It may be assumed that this condition obtains when both orifices of the double microelectrode are in the extracellular tissue of the spinal cord. Under such conditions the recorded potential is directly proportional to the applied current, which is to be expected for a coupling resistance that is independent of current flow. As measured in this way the coupling resistance usually has been about 200,000 Ω (cf. line of open circles of Figure 21C), but with different electrodes there have been widely differing values, which presumably depend on the effectiveness with which the partition separates the orifices of the double microelectrode.

For any given current a much larger potential is recorded when the double microelectrode is implanted in a motoneurone, i.e., there is a large additional resistance common to the current-applying and voltage-recording circuits. Since there is reason to believe that the specific resistivity of neuronal cytoplasm is very little larger than that of extracellular fluids, only a negligible fraction of this additional resistance is attributable to an increased coupling resistance; hence virtually all of it must occur across the neuronal membrane. Within limits the membrane resistance so measured was independent of the current intensity, as is shown by the linear relationship of measured potential to applied current (Figures 4, 21C, filled circles), and it was surprising to find that the resistance was virtually the same for depolarizing and hyperpolariz-

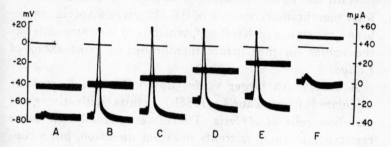

Figure 4

A series of six responses of a motoneurone evoked by an antidromic impulse, and recorded through one barrel of a double microelectrode. In *C*, no extrinsic current was applied and the spike response rises from the resting potential of −65 mV to a crest at +18 mV. In *B* and *A*, the membrane was hyperpolarized by a current through the other barrel of the microelectrode, which in A was sufficient to block the antidromic invasion (cf. Fig. 18A). In *D*, *E*, and *F*, the membrane was depolarized by a current, and in F antidromic invasion was also blocked. All records are formed by superposition of about forty faint traces. The intensities of the applied currents are signalled by the records seen as simple horizontal lines, the current scale being on the right. Potential scale is on the left, zero potential difference across the membrane being indicated by the horizontal lines drawn at about the level of zero on the potential scale. The level is strictly at zero on the scale only for record C. The small deviations for other records arise because of the potential drop in the coupling resistance as determined in extracellular records which are not shown. Note that the initial levels of the voltage traces move in parallel with the levels of the respective current traces, i.e., there is a linear relationship.

ing currents (Coombs *et al.*, 1955a). In this respect the neuronal membrane is very different from the membranes of giant axons, which have a much lower resistance for depolarizing currents (Cole and Curtis, 1941; Hodgkin, Huxley, and Katz, 1952). On the other hand, the membrane of mammalian muscle fibres resembles that of motoneurones in showing no appreciable rectification (Boyd and Martin, 1956). With different neurones, values ranging from 0.4 MΩ to 1.3 MΩ have been obtained for the membrane resistance, 0.8 MΩ being a reasonable value for a standard neurone in good condition (Coombs *et al.*, 1955a; Frank and Fuortes, 1956b).

With an effective neuronal surface of $5 \times 10^{-4} cm^2$, a total membrane resistance of 0.8 MΩ gives a specific membrane resistance of $400 \ \Omega \ cm^2$, which is of the same order as the values for the surface membranes of giant axons of *Loligo*.

A very much larger value (up to $10^5 \ \Omega \ cm^2$) may be calculated from Tauc's (1955b) results with the giant ganglion cells of *Aplysia*. There was virtually the same resistance to small currents in either direction, but a considerable rectification occurred with large currents.

By a bridge technique Araki and Otani (1955) have determined the membrane resistance of toad motoneurones that were impaled by a single microelectrode. The values so obtained were considerably higher (3.0 MΩ to 5.8 MΩ), from which a mean specific membrane resistance of $270 \ \Omega \ cm^2$ was calculated on the basis of a very low estimate ($6 \times 10^{-5} \ cm^2$) for the membrane area.

The attempt to determine membrane resistance with depolarizations of more than from 10 mV to 15 mV is complicated by the repetitive generation of impulses by the motoneurone. This discharge usually has ceased within a few seconds and the measurements then have been made. When the microelectrode is filled by a potassium salt, this procedure is justified because further continuance of the current produces no significant change in the measured potential, and hence in the computed membrane resistance. Also, when the depolarization is too small to generate impulses, the membrane resistance shows no significant change after the first measurement, which can be made a few milliseconds after the application of the current. Observations under these conditions are of special interest, since they show that, when uncomplicated by impulse discharges, the motoneuronal membrane differs basically from the membrane of giant axons in that its membrane resistance is not lowered on account of an increased potassium conductance that is produced by a subthreshold depolarization (cf. Cole and Curtis, 1941; Hodgkin, Huxley, and Katz, 1952; Hodgkin and Huxley, 1952a,b).

Depletion of intracellular potassium is the only ionic change which has been found to have any significant effect on the membrane conductance (Coombs *et al.*, 1955a). After a large injection of sodium or tetramethylammonium ions, there is a decrease by as much as 40 per cent, and there is a slow recovery after the sodium injection. This decrease is explicable if the membrane conductance is attributable largely to K^+ ions, because they will be depleted by the injection of these other cations. Thus we have to assume that the motoneuronal membrane resembles that of giant axons in having a high resting conductance for K^+ ions, but differs from it in that this conductance is not increased by depolarization.

3. The Electric Time Constant of the Neuronal Membrane

If a rectangular current pulse (I) is applied to the simple network of Figure 5A, having a resistance (R) in parallel with a condenser (C), the potential across the con-

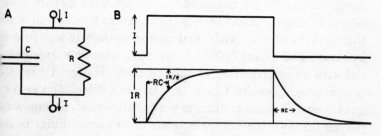

Figure 5

A. Simple electrical network of condenser C in parallel with resistance R, a current, I, being passed between the two terminals as shown. *B.* Upper drawing shows time course of a rectangular current pulse of intensity, I. Lower drawing shows on the same time scale the potential recorded between the two terminals. Further description in text.

denser will increase exponentially to a value that is given by the IR product (Figure 5B). The time course of this exponential increase, as specified by the time to approach 1/e of the final value, i.e., IR/e, is given by the RC product, which is called the electric time constant of the system. On cessation of the current the potential across the condenser decays with a similar time course.

The surface membranes of giant axons and of muscle fibres have been shown to approximate such a simple electrical system (cf. Katz, 1948; Hodgkin, 1951), with time constants ranging from 1 msec. to 30 msec., so it is likely that the surface membrane covering the soma, dendrites, and initial axonal segment of the motoneurone would exhibit similar properties. The most direct method of determining the time constant for a motoneurone would be to record with an intracellular microelectrode the time course of the potential generated by the passage of a rectangular current pulse through that electrode. Unfortunately, the neuronal membrane usually has a resistance of less than 10 per cent of the electrode resistance, so the total observed potential change will be dominated by the electrode properties. If the assumption be made that the electrode properties are not altered during the passage of a current, the steady potential due to the IR product for the electrode and other resistances in series with the neuronal membrane could be balanced out by a bridge circuit. The potential change could then be assumed to be due solely to the membrane, and with toad motoneurones it was found by Araki and Otani (1955) to be approximately exponential with a time constant of about 4 msec. (range, 1.5 msec. to 8 msec.). Coombs, Curtis and Eccles (1956a), however, have found that, in control experiments when current was passed through the microelectrode in an extracellular position, it often did not behave as a simple resistance. At the onset and cessation of the current there was an exponential change having a time course resembling that recorded intracellularly, but being of much smaller magnitude (Figure 6E). Furthermore, reversal of current sometimes

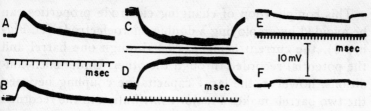

Figure 6

A and *B* show intracellularly recorded excitatory postsynaptic potentials which are generated monosynaptically by a single volley. Intracellular potential change in a positive direction is shown as an upward deflection. In *C* and *D*, hyperpolarizing and depolarizing rectangular current pulses of 8.5 x $10^{-9}A$ were applied through the single microelectrode used for *A* and *B*. Note change in time scales. A resistance capacitance network was employed in order to give approximate compensation for all potential changes occurring in the system apart from those on the cell membrane. In *E* and *F,* the same current was applied through the electrode immediately after withdrawing from the cell, the amplification being the same as in *A, C,* and *D,* but with slower time course. The relatively small potential changes occurring after the first millisecond in *E* and *F* have to be subtracted from those similarly occurring in *C* and *D,* respectively, in order to determine the potential time course for the cell membrane. Records formed by superposition of about forty faint traces (Coombs, Curtis, and Eccles, 1956a).

did not give a mirror-image change in the recorded potential as reported by Araki and Otani (1955). It appears that our microelectrodes changed their electrical properties during the passage of current, which was also observed by Frank and Fuortes (1956b). Such an effect would be expected to arise because of both the ionic migration caused by the current and the interaction of ions with the glass surface at the most constricted part of the microelectrode (R. H. Adrian, 1956). The best approximation that could be obtained was to record the potential-time courses produced by currents applied in both directions intracellularly (Figure 6C,D), and then repeat the observations immediately after withdrawal from the motoneurone (Figure 6E,F). The differences between the two series of curves were assumed to be due to the motoneuronal membrane, which in this manner was observed to have a time constant of about 2.5 msec. (range 2 msec. to 4 msec.) for motoneurones in good condition.

This complication of changing electrode properties can be avoided by employing a double microelectrode (cf. Figure 3), the current being passed through one barrel and the potential recorded through the other. Under such conditions, however, the large capacitative coupling between the two barrels makes a major contribution to the recorded potential for the first few milliseconds after the onset or cessation of the current (cf. Figures 16, 25A). With the double electrode in an extracellular position, however, it is possible virtually to eliminate this artefact by a reactance bridge (Figure 7E,F). Since it is justifiable to assume that

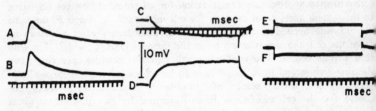

Figure 7

Double microelectrode with potentials recorded through one barrel and currents applied through the other. *A* and *B* are excitatory postsynaptic potentials generated monosynaptically, the presynaptic volley being a little below maximum strength in *A*. *C* and *D* show potentials generated by rectangular current pulses of 12.5×10^{-9}A which are in the hyperpolarizing and depolarizing directions respectively. As shown in the extracellular records, *E* and *F*, the compensating network virtually eliminated all changes in potential, except those within 1 msec. after the onset and cessation of the pulses. The currents in *E* and *F* were 16×10^{-9}A in the hyperpolarizing and depolarizing directions respectively (Coombs, Curtis, and Eccles 1956a).

the intracellular position of the microelectrode differs only by the addition of the neuronal membrane to the circuits the intracellular records (Figure 7C,D) will then give the actual time course of the membrane potential change that is produced by the onset and cessation of a rectangular current pulse. The time constant of the motoneuronal membrane as directly determined in this manner has also been about 2.5 msec. (Coombs, Curtis and Eccles, 1956a).

Tauc (1955b) has been able virtually to eliminate the

coupling between the current and potential circuits by introducing two independent microelectrodes into the giant ganglion cells of *Aplysia*. The electric time constant was observed to be as long as 150 msec.

An indirect method for determining the time constant of the motoneuronal membrane has depended on experimental evidence which indicated that the excitatory and inhibitory postsynaptic potentials were generated by ionic fluxes that traversed the subsynaptic membrane for no more than 2 msec. (Brock, Coombs, and Eccles, 1952b; J. C. Eccles, 1952; Coombs, Eccles, and Fatt, 1955c,d). In that event the observed exponential decay of these postsynaptic potentials would have the time constant of the motoneuronal membrane, which in this way was determined to be about 4 msec. The methods of direct measurement, however, show that this value is in error by a factor of almost two. The decay of the postsynaptic potentials is slowed by a small residuum of synaptic activity, as is illustrated in Figure 11A, and it was incorrect to assume that the active phase of transmitter action had ceased after 2 msec.

With the crustacean stretch receptor cells, inhibitory impulses produce a postsynaptic potential which declines exponentially with a time constant of 15 msec. to 20 msec. (Kuffler and Eyzaguirre, 1955). Since there is good evidence that the active inhibitory process continues for at least 20 msec. (cf. Chapter III), the time constant of the membrane must likewise be briefer than is indicated by the exponential decay of the inhibitory synaptic potential. It cannot be much briefer, however, for there is a similar slow decay of the soma potential that is produced when an antidromic impulse fails to invade (Eyzaguirre and Kuffler, 1955b), so probably a value of 15 msec. is not far in error.

4. The Capacitance of the Neuronal Membrane

The capacitance of the surface membrane of a standard mammalian motoneurone may be calculated by dividing the time constant (2.5×10^{-3} sec.) by the resistance (8×10^{5} Ω), a value of about 3×10^{-9}F being so obtained. The specific membrane capacitance is obtained by dividing this value by the effective area of the membrane (5×10^{-4} cm^2), the value of 6 μF/cm^2 being much higher than with the membrane of giant axons (Hodgkin, 1951), but surface membranes of some muscle fibres have higher specific capacitances (Fatt and Katz, 1951; 1953). Possibly the effective area of the membrane has been underestimated. With doubling of the area, the specific resistance would be increased to 800Ω cm^2, and the specific capacitance reduced to 3 μF/cm^2. From their determinations of membrane resistance and time constant for toad motoneurones, Araki and Otani (1955) calculate a capacitance of about 1×10^{-9}F, and a specific membrane capacitance of 17.5 μF/cm^2. With giant ganglion cells of *Aplysia* a value of from 1.5 to 3 μF/cm^2 may be calculated for the specific membrane capacitance (Tauc, 1955b). Unfortunately, the available data are insufficient for the assessment of the capacitances of other neuronal membranes.

5. *Discussion*

In the study of synaptic action on a nerve cell, it will emerge that both the generation of impulses by excitatory synaptic action and their prevention by inhibitory synaptic action are fully explicable by the changes produced in the postsynaptic membrane potential. Thus specially privileged information is provided by intracellular recording. The exterior of a nerve cell remains virtually isopotential with the indifferent grounded electrode, while the whole interior of the soma is practically at a uniform potential. Hence the intracellularly recorded potential provides a reliable measure of the potential changes across the soma membrane.

In attempting to explain the behaviour of a nerve cell under all manner of experimental conditions, we may regard it simply as a small globule bounded by the surface membrane and containing a salt solution very different from the external medium. Values for the volume and surface area of this globule have been derived above for the motoneurone and the measurements of the voltage, resistance, electric time constant, and capacitance have been described. Investigations on giant axons (Cole and Curtis, 1939; Hodgkin, Huxley, and Katz, 1952) have shown that the membrane capacitance suffers virtually no change during the profound alteration in membrane properties that occurs during an impulse, the changes in membrane potential being brought about by flux of ions across the surface membrane. It is therefore justifiable to assume, at least provisionally, that changes in the membrane potential of nerve cells are entirely attributable to ionic movements across the surface membrane. It will emerge that on the basis of this provisional assumption satisfactory explanations can be developed for all the potential changes observed with intracellular recording from nerve cells.

With a motoneurone the external saline medium may be assumed to be simply an ultra-filtrate of blood with the composition shown in Table 1, which gives the mean values for an ultra-filtrate of cat blood (cf. Coombs et al., 1955b, pp. 361-62). It will be helpful at this stage to anticipate some of the later conclusions about the ionic composition of the motoneurone (Chapters II, III). These conclusions conform in general with results obtained with giant axons which can be investigated in isolation and which are particularly suitable for investigation by radioactive tracers. The values that are given in Table 1 are for the concentration of free ions, but there is evidence that ions are not bound to any appreciable extent in giant axons (Hodgkin and Keynes, 1953; Caldwell, 1955).

The internal concentrations of K^+ and Cl^- ions are determined by calculation according to the Nernst equation from values for the external concentrations and the respective equilibrium potentials of -90 mV and -70 mV (cf. Chapters II and III). The internal concentration of Na^+ ions is more uncertain, but the maximum size of the spike

TABLE 1. *Ionic concentrations and equilibrium potentials for cat motoneurones*

	outside mM	inside mM	equilibrium potential (according to the Nernst equation) in mV
Na	150	about 15	about +60
K	5.5	150	−90
Cl	125	9	−70

potential suggests a value of the order shown, which is in general accord with the 1 to 10 ratio observed with giant axons (Hodgkin, 1951; Keynes and Lewis, 1951), though recently a high value (40 mM) has been reported for intracellular sodium of medullated axons with a consequent ratio as low as 1 to 6 across the membrane (Krnjevic, 1955).

It is generally agreed that the movements of ions across surface membranes occur by two distinct mechanisms. With one mechanism the ions move freely by diffusion, the net movement for an ion species across unit area of a membrane being governed by the permeability of the membrane to that species and the electrochemical gradient for that species. With the other mechanism the ions of a species are forced to move against their electrochemical gradient, i.e., thermodynamically they are pumped uphill, a process which involves work which ultimately must be derived from metabolic energy. Since the concepts of electrochemical gradient, electrochemical potential, and equilibrium potential are to be used extensively in the ensuing discussions, it is proposed to discuss these concepts in relation to illustrative examples.

In crossing the surface membrane inward the negatively charged Cl⁻ ions have to travel "uphill" along an electrical gradient, i.e., from a positively charged to a negatively charged surface. Conversely, the movement of Cl⁻ ions in the other direction would have an equivalent "drive" from the gradient, i.e., the ions travel along a downhill gradient

It would be expected that with equal concentrations on the two sides the numbers of ions traversing the membrane uphill (inward) would be much smaller than those traversing the membrane downhill (outward). However, by increasing the concentration of Cl⁻ ions outside, and hence the number of attempted inward traverses, this discrepancy can be diminished. The numbers of Cl⁻ ions traversing the membrane in the two directions are exactly equal when the relative concentration between inside and outside, $\dfrac{Cl_i}{Cl_o}$, is related to the membrane potential, E_{Cl} (in mV), by the Nernst equation (at 38°C),

$$E_{Cl} = 61.5 \log_{10} \frac{Cl_i}{Cl_o}$$

Thus a steady state then obtains for Cl⁻ ions, E_{Cl} being the equilibrium potential for Cl⁻ ions when there is this relative concentration across the membrane. We can further say that, at the equilibrium potential for any ion species, there is zero electrochemical gradient across the membrane. The experimental evidence of Chapter III indicates that, for a normal motoneurone, $E_{Cl} = -70$ mV, i.e., that Cl⁻ ions are in electrochemical equilibrium at the normal resting potential, there being, in accordance with the Nernst equation, a fourteen fold difference in concentration to compensate for the potential difference of −70 mV (cf. Table 1). If the difference in concentration were less (say only seven fold), then the equilibrium potential as derived from the Nernst equation would be only −52 mV and there would be across the membrane an outward electrochemical gradient of about 18 mV for Cl⁻ ions. We might then say that at a membrane potential of −70 mV there is an electrochemical potential of +18 mV for Cl⁻ ions.

Experimental evidence given in Chapter II indicates that the value of E_K (the equilibrium potential for K⁺ ions) is normally about −90 mV. Thus at a resting potential of −70 mV there will be an electrochemical potential of −20 mV for K⁺ ions. The value for K_i of 150 mM is

approximately twice that required for diffusional equilibrium at the resting membrane potential. Thus at the
resting potential of −70 mV the outward diffusional flux
of K⁺ ions would be twice as great as the inward. A steady

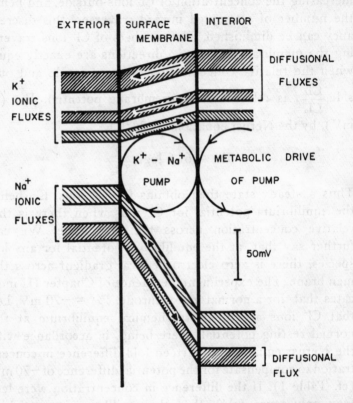

Figure 8

Diagrammatic representation of K⁺ and Na⁺ fluxes through the surface
membrane in the resting state. The slopes in the flux channels across the
membrane represent the respective electrochemical gradients. At the resting
membrane potential (−70 mV) the electrochemical gradients, as drawn for
the K⁺ and Na⁺ ions, correspond respectively to potentials which are 20 mV
more positive and about 130 mV more negative than the equilibrium potentials (note the potential scale). The fluxes due to diffusion and the operation of the pump are distinguished by the direction of hatching. The outward diffusional flux of Na⁺ ions would be less than 1 per cent of the
inward and so is too insignificant to be indicated as a separate channel in
this diagram, because the magnitudes of the fluxes are indicated by the
widths of the respective channels.

state can be maintained only if the deficiency in inward flux is made up by an inward pumping mechanism which must for this purpose operate to give an inward ionic flux of the same magnitude as that due to diffusion. The conditions may be shown diagrammatically in Figure 8, where the electrochemical potential of 20 mV is shown, and the widths of the channels denote the relative magnitudes of the fluxes.

The diagram of Figure 8 may be completed by adding the Na^+ fluxes. At the resting membrane potential the electrochemical potential for Na^+ ions is in the opposite direction to K^+ and much larger (approximately 130 mV). As a consequence, the inward diffusional flux would be over one hundred times the outward, so that, as illustrated, a steady state is attained when the outward pumping of Na^+ virtually equals the inward diffusion. Reasons are given in Chapter III for assuming that, as with giant axons (Hodgkin and Keynes, 1955), the inward pumping of K^+ ions is coupled, as shown, with the outward pumping of Na^+ ions.

Since the membrane of a standard motoneurone has a capacitance of about 3×10^{-9}F and a potential of -70 mV (7×10^{-2}V), it will have an internal charge of 2.1×10^{-10} coulombs, which corresponds to an excess of about 2×10^{-15} equiv. of anions inside the motoneurone. It may be assumed that this excess of anions is maintained as a steady state by virtue of the operation of the coupled $Na^+ - K^+$ pump. It is seen in Table 1 that Cl^- ions account for a relatively small fraction of the total internal ions. The main anion constitution of nerve cells remains unknown. With the giant axons of *Loligo* the principal internal anion is isethionate (Koechlin, 1954). This anion, however, does not appear to be in a significant concentration in other giant axons. Glutamate, fumarate and aspartate also account for some of the anion fraction (cf. Lewis, 1952). The effect of anoxia in causing a rapid fall in membrane potential of nerve cells (van Harreveld, 1946; Lloyd, 1953) is probably attributable to the failure of the $Na^+ - K^+$

pump to maintain the anion excess as the metabolism declines.

The activity of the coupled sodium-potassium pump is not significantly modified by alteration of the membrane potential of giant axons (Hodgkin and Keynes, 1955), but it seems that it is potentiated by increase in the internal sodium concentration, as also occurs with motoneurones (cf. Chapter III). Thus ultimately the membrane potential would be set by the effectiveness with which the internal sodium concentration drives the pump and by the concentration of the fixed internal anions. As a consequence of their experiments on microinjection of ions into giant axons, Grundfest, Kao, and Altamirano (1954) likewise have postulated that the activity of the sodium pump determines the membrane potential. When, as probably occurs with chloride ions, diffusion alone controls the movement across the membrane, such ion species can contribute nothing to a steady membrane potential. Ultimately their distribution will be related to the membrane potential in accordance with the Nernst equilibrium equation, but they can play no part in determining that potential.

The diffusional ionic exchange across the membrane, however, is of great significance in relation to transient changes of membrane potential. Such conditions do not appreciably change the activity of the sodium-potassium pump (Hodgkin and Keynes, 1955), but they profoundly affect the diffusional exchange. Thus the diffusional exchange of ions alone would contribute to the membrane resistance as measured above. Furthermore, if the membrane potential is displaced from its steady-state value (the resting potential), the diffusional ionic fluxes are unbalanced so that the steady-state value tends to be restored, and, on cessation of the disturbing influence, they restore the resting potential with a time course corresponding to the electric time constant of the membrane.

The measured membrane resistance of a motoneurone (about $8 \times 10^5 \Omega$) may be expressed as a conductance of about 1.2×10^{-6} mhos. As with giant axons (Hodgkin and Huxley, 1952b) and probably muscle fibres (Keynes, 1954), this conductance appears to be largely a potassium conductance. No measurement of potassium conductance has been possible with motoneurones. An approximate estimate of 0.25×10^{-6} mhos., however, has been made for the chloride conductance (Chapter III), which is approximately the same fraction of the total as has been observed for giant axons (Hodgkin and Huxley, 1952b).

In final summary, the electrical properties of the surface membrane of the standard motoneurone may be represented by the formal electrical diagram of Figure 9.

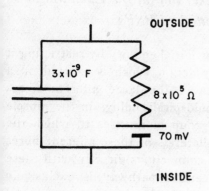

OUTSIDE

3×10^{-9} F

8×10^{5} Ω

70 mV

INSIDE

Figure 9

Formal electrical diagram of the resting membrane of a standard motoneurone, showing mean values for the membrane potential, capacitance, and resistance.

CHAPTER II

THE EXCITATORY REACTIONS
OF NERVE CELLS

A. MOTONEURONES

1. Intracellular Recording of the Excitatory Postsynaptic Potential (EPSP)

We will simplify our initial enquiry by restricting it to the synaptic excitatory action which is exerted on a motoneurone by impulses in the large afferent fibres (Group Ia) from the annulospiral endings in the muscle spindles of the synergic group of muscles to which the motoneurone belongs. Collaterals of these afferent fibres make excitatory synaptic connections directly with these motoneurones, i.e., the central pathway is exclusively monosynaptic. Initially, also, only those excitatory synaptic actions which are uncomplicated by spike potentials will be considered. However, so far as they have been investigated (cf. Woodbury and Patton, 1952; J. C. Eccles, 1953; Araki and Otani, 1955; Frank and Fuortes, 1955a,b) polysynaptic excitatory actions on motoneurones appear to be due essentially to a depolarization that is produced by the same type of synaptic action. The discharge of impulses is evoked at about the same level of depolarization. Thus the only difference appears to arise because of the asynchronous and repetitive synaptic bombardment.

As shown in the three records of Figure 10A–C, a single presynaptic volley generates a depolarizing potential, the excitatory postsynaptic potential (EPSP), that runs virtually the same time course regardless of volley size. This

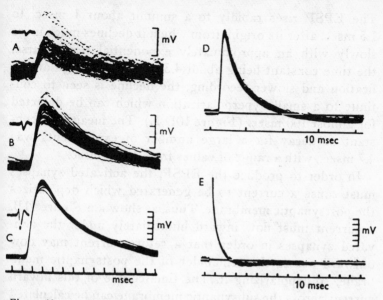

Figure 10

A–C. EPSP's obtained in a biceps-semitendinosus motoneurone with
afferent volleys of different size. Inset records at the left of main records
show afferent volley recorded near entry of dorsal nerve roots into spinal
cord. They are taken with negativity downward and at a constant amplification for which no scale is given. Records of EPSP are taken at an amplification that decreases in steps from *A* to *C* as the response increases.
Separate vertical scales are given for each record of EPSP. All records
formed by superposition of about forty faint traces. *D, E.* Same EPSP
as in Figure 10C, but at slower sweep speeds. A base line is drawn through
the initial level of potential (Coombs *et al.,* 1955c).

observation indicates that each excitatory synapse generates a potential change of this same time course, and
that the recorded potentials of Figure 10 are produced by
a simple summation of these elemental synaptic potentials.
Thus Figure 10 provides an illustration of the classical concept of spatial summation (Sherrington, 1925; 1929).

With monosynaptic excitatory action the EPSP can
first be detected about 0.5 msec. after the primary afferent
volley has entered the spinal cord, this instant being signaled in the inset records of Figure 10 by the first reversal
point of the triphasic spike potentials from the dorsal root.

The EPSP rises rapidly to a summit about 1 msec. to 1.5 msec. after its origin, from which it declines much more slowly with an approximately exponential time course, the time constant being about 4.3 msec. With high amplification and slower recording, the decline is seen to continue to a small hyperpolarization which can be detected for almost 100 msec. (Figure 10D,E). The mean time constant of decay for a large number of experiments was 4.7 msec., with a range of values from 4 to 7 msec.

In order to produce the EPSP, the activated synapses must cause a current to be generated which depolarizes the postsynaptic membrane. Thus, as shown in Figure 11B, a current must flow inward immediately under the activated synapses in order that a return current may flow outward across the remainder of the postsynaptic membrane, so depolarizing it. The time course of this inward current across the subsynaptic membrane can be calculated for those motoneurones whose electric time constants have been measured directly (cf. Figures 6, 7). For example, the motoneurone giving the EPSP's of Figure 6A,B had a time constant of 2.5 msec. (cf. Figure 6C,D) and the calculated time course of the generating current is shown by the broken line in Figure 11A (Coombs, Curtis and Eccles, 1956a). Typically, as in Figure 11A, this current rises steeply to a maximum in about 0.5 msec. from its onset and then rapidly declines for about 1 msec. (cf. Figure 23E), but it is still about 10 per cent of its maximum at 2 msec., and thereafter it slowly declines for many milliseconds. This residuum of the current causes the EPSP to decay with a time constant (4.3 msec.) that is much longer than that of the membrane. The nature of this current through the subsynaptic membrane will be considered later. Full consideration also will be given later (Chapter V) to the transmitter substance that is assumed to be liberated from the presynaptic terminals and to be instrumental in producing the effective change in the subsynaptic membrane.

In a previous attempt to determine the time course of the subsynaptic current that generated the monosynaptic

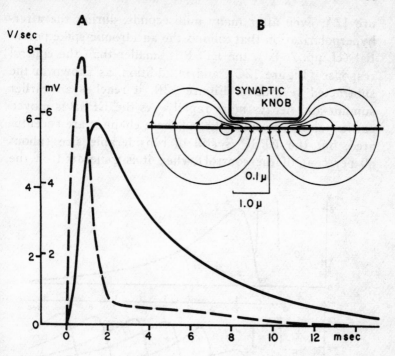

Figure 11

A. The continuous line is the mean of several monosynaptic EPSP's that were photographed just before the records of Figure 6, while the broken line shows the time course of the subsynaptic current required to generate this potential change. If the membrane capacity is assumed to be constant at (say) 3×10^{-9}F, the V/sec. scale becomes a current scale, 2V/sec. being equivalent to 6×10^{-9}A and so on. The time constant of the membrane, 2.5 msec., is derived from Figures 6C–F. *B.* Diagram showing an activated excitatory synaptic knob and the postsynaptic membrane. As indicated by the scales for distance, the synaptic cleft is shown at 10 times the scale for width as against length. The current generating the EPSP passes in through the cleft and inward across the activated subsynaptic membrane, but outward across the remainder of the postsynaptic membrane (Coombs, *et al.,* 1956a).

EPSP, an impulse was caused to propagate over the surface of the motoneurone at various times relative to the EPSP (Brock *et al.,* 1952b; J. C. Eccles, 1953; Coombs *et al.,* 1955c). The simplest situation is provided if this impulse is generated by antidromic invasion of the soma dendrites to give the SD spike potential. As shown in Figure 12A, even after many milliseconds, during the after-hyperpolarization that follows the antidromic spike potential (cf. pp. 76-83), the EPSP is smaller than the control response (Figure 12C), and in addition, as shown in the subtracted records of Figure 12B, it reaches an earlier summit and decays more rapidly. As the EPSP is moved earlier relative to the spike, all these changes are accentuated, but the EPSP is still of considerable size (about 30 per cent of the control) when it is generated on the

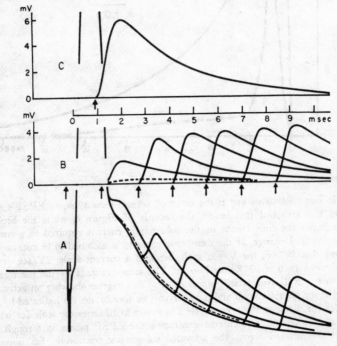

Figure 12

A. Combined tracing of the motoneurone action potential alone (spike and after-potential) and the action potential with monosynaptic EPSP's superimposed on it at various times from its onset. Broken line is response to a presynaptic volley that would set up an EPSP beginning at the first arrow of Figure 12B. *B.* EPSP's set up at various times during an action potential, obtained by subtracting the control action potential from the superimposed action potential and EPSP's shown in *A.* *C.* Isolated EPSP obtained in the absence of action potential. Note that the spike potential of *A* is shown by interrupted lines extending up through *B* and *C.*

later part of the falling phase of the spike, at the second arrow of Figure 12B. However, when the presynaptic volley is timed so that it would set up an EPSP at the first arrow (about 1.5 msec. earlier), there is only the very small response shown by the broken-line curves (Coombs, Curtis and Eccles, 1956a).

On the basis of similar observations it was concluded that the synaptic mechanism is not able to generate any appreciable EPSP if it is prevented from doing so for 1.2 msec.; and hence that the EPSP is generated by a mechanism whose depolarizing activity persists for no longer than about 1.2 msec. (Coombs et al., 1955c). It was too readily assumed, on analogy with the amphibian end plate potential (Kuffler, 1942; Fatt and Katz, 1951), that the exponential decays of the monosynaptic EPSP and the directly evoked IPSP were due to a single factor, the time constant of the motoneuronal membrane, which was thus shown to be about 4 msec. The interaction experiments with the antidromic spike potential were regarded as confirmatory of this simple concept, because, after the very short duration so indicated for the active depolarizing current (cf. Figure 12), the time course of the membrane potential would be governed solely by the electric time constant of the membrane.

It may now be asked: How can these results with antidromic interaction be reconciled with the much longer time course of the active depolarizing current shown in Figure 11A? The time course of the excitatory current, as given by the broken line of Figure 11A, enables an approximate calculation to be made of the relative sizes of the EPSP's that would be predicted for the two shortest test intervals in Figure 12. It appears that the subsynaptic current is not effective in building up an EPSP until it is late on the declining phase of the spike potential. At the second shortest test interval in Figure 12A the maximum subsynaptic current operated at this earliest effective stage after the spike. On the other hand, at the shortest test interval the subsynaptic current was 1.5 msec. earlier relative to the spike and so would have declined to a low level (cf. Figure 11A) before it had a chance to be effective. At the most it would then have been 10 per cent to 15 per cent of its maximum, and the EPSP which it added is seen to be correspondingly smaller than the EPSP added at the second shortest test interval (cf. the broken line of Figure 12A). Hitherto it has been assumed that these small effects were due to the delayed action of polysynaptic excitatory pathways. It will now be realized that the causal agent is provided by the slowly declining residuum of the active depolarizing current which is generated by a monosynaptic excitatory action (cf. Figure 11A).

It can be concluded that it is merely fortuitous that the EPSP decays exponentially with a time constant of 4 msec. to 7 msec. A passive decay would be more rapid with a time constant of about 2.5 msec. (the electric time constant of the membrane), but it is delayed by the small residuum of active depolarizing current as illustrated in Figure 11A (Coombs, Curtis and Eccles, 1956a).

2. Extracellular Recording of Synaptic Excitatory Action

There is general agreement that, when the recording microelectrode lies outside of the cell in a motor nucleus, a volley having excitatory synaptic activity generates, relative to an indifferent electrode, a diphasic spike potential in positive-negative sequence, closely followed by a more prolonged negative potential wave, as in Figure 13 at a depth of 4.1 mm. There is general agreement also that the diphasic spike is generated by the primary afferent volley as it approaches and then reaches the presynaptic terminals in the nucleus. However, the later negative wave has been attributed on the one hand to a prolonged negativity of the presynaptic terminals (Renshaw, 1946b; Lloyd and McIntyre, 1949; Lloyd, 1952a; 1955) and on the other hand to the postsynaptic currents that generate the

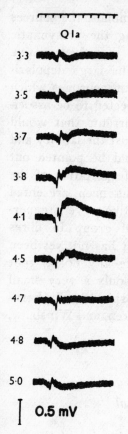

Q Ia

3.3

3.5

3.7

3.8

4.1

4.5

4.7

4.8

5.0

0.5 mV

Figure 13

Microelectrode records of the focal potentials generated by a group Ia volley in quadriceps nerve, electrode negativity being recorded upward. The potentials are recorded successively along a track passing through the ventral horn in L6 segment. The numbers give the depths in millimetres from the dorsal surface of the cord at which the responses were recorded. The quadriceps motor nucleus is centered on 4.1 mm depth. Time in msec. (Eccles, Fatt, Landgren, and Winsbury, 1954).

EPSP and cause its electrotonic spread along the motor axons (Brooks and Eccles, 1947b; J. C. Eccles, 1950: Brock *et al.*, 1952a). It is possible to decide between these two conflicting interpretations by locating the source of the currents that flow into the sink in the motoneurone nucleus.

Figure 13 illustrates a general observation that, on a dorsoventral track through the motoneurone nucleus, the sources for its prolonged negative potential are located only on the ventral side of the nucleus along the motor axon pathway, as is shown at 4.8 mm. and 5.0 mm. by the positive potential wave of similar time course. If the negative wave

were generated in the presynaptic terminals, the sources
would lie dorsally, i.e., upstream along the presynaptic
fibres. It may, therefore, be concluded that the negative
wave is generated postsynaptically. The large depolarization of the soma and dendrites of motoneurones which
occurs during the EPSP would be expected to be associated with the flow of extracellular currents that would
give an extracellular potential having just the latency and
time course that is observed. It should be pointed out
further that, apart from the above interpretation of the
negative wave, no other evidence has been presented
which would indicate that a slow negative wave is generated by the presynaptic terminals of group Ia fibres
in the motoneurone nucleus. In fact, it has not yet been
shown that group Ia volleys generate any dorsal root
potential. Furthermore, they produce only a very small
potential on the dorsal surface of the spinal cord (Bernhard, 1952b; 1953; Eccles, Fatt, Landgren, and Winsbury,
1954).

3. Relationship of the EPSP
to the Generation of a Spike Potential

As shown in Figure 14, increasing the size of the primary afferent volley not only increases the size of the
EPSP (as in Figure 10), but it also may cause the motoneurone to generate a spike potential, i.e., to discharge an
impulse. The latency of this discharge is progressively
shortened as the EPSP is increased (Figure 14B–F). It
appears that, just as with giant axons (Hodgkin, Huxley,
and Katz, 1952; Hodgkin and Huxley, 1952c), when the
membrane potential is diminished below a critical level, a
self-regenerative process of increased sodium conductance
with the consequent inward movement of Na^+ ions causes
a rapid depolarization running on even to reversal of the
membrane potential. There is general agreement that this
discharge is due to spatial summation within the moto-

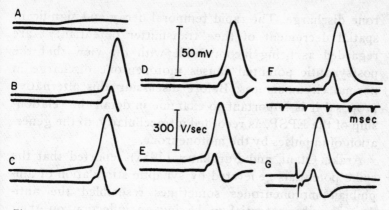

Figure 14

A–F. Intracellular potentials generated in a motoneurone by a mono-synaptic excitatory volley. This volley is increased progressively in size from *A* to *F*, with the consequence that the EPSP is larger, and in *B* to *F* the spike potential is generated progressively earlier. The spike is always initiated when the EPSP attains approximately the same voltage (6 mV in *B* to *F*). *G* shows that a similar spike potential is produced when an anti-dromic impulse invades the motoneurone. An electrically differentiated record of each potential wave lies immediately below it. Note the correspond-ing scale in V/sec. Further description in text. (Coombs, Curtis, and Eccles, 1956b).

neurone of the excitatory effects of many synapses. This spatial summation may be explained simply by the summa-tion of the EPSP's produced by the individual synapses so that the depolarization reaches the threshold level for generating a propagating impulse (Barron and Matthews, 1938; Bremer, Bonnet, and Moldaver, 1942; Eccles, 1946a; Brooks and Eccles, 1947b; Fessard and Posternak, 1950; Bremer, 1951; 1953a; Fatt, 1954; Brock *et al.*, 1952a; Coombs *et al.*, 1955c). However, a recent series of investi-gations (Lloyd and McIntyre, 1955; Hunt, 1955) has led to the conclusion "that the postsynaptic potential is not an essential step leading to monosynaptic reflex trans-mission." As a consequence it has been postulated that monosynaptic excitatory impulses are effective in evoking motoneuronal discharge by a "transmitter potentiality" which can be assessed solely by the criterion of motoneurone discharge. The rapid temporal decay and significant spatial decrement of the "transmitter potentiality" are regarded as being incompatible with the view that the postsynaptic potential causes motoneurone discharge in normal circumstances. Before discussing this alternative proposal it is important to examine in detail the relationship of the EPSP, as recorded intracellularly, to the generation of impulses by the motoneurone.

Araki, Otani, and Furukawa (1953) reported that the spike potentials generated by synaptic stimulation of amphibian motoneurones sometimes resembled the antidromic spike potential in having an inflection on their rising phase. With faster recording Frank and Fuortes (1956b) regularly observed that, when generated synaptically, the spike potential did not have a smooth rising phase as originally described (Brock *et al.*, 1952a), but was interrupted by a very slight notch, which occurred at much the same potential (30 mV to 40 mV) as was observed with the much more pronounced notch on the rising phase of the spike generated by antidromic invasion (Figures 14G, 18A, 26A; Brock *et al.*, 1952a; 1953). Independent confirmation has been provided by Fatt (1956b)

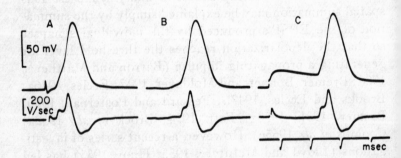

Figure 15

A, B, and C, respectively, show the intracellular potentials produced when a spike response of a motoneurone is generated antidromically, synaptically (monosynaptic), and by a directly applied current (by a double electrode). An electrically differentiated record of each potential wave lies immediately below it. Note that there is an inflection at approximately the same level (about 30 mV) on the rising phases of the three spikes (Fatt, 1956b).

and Coombs, Curtis and Eccles (1956b), who greatly accentuated the effect by recording the rising phase with electrical differentiation (Figure 15A,B). The significance of this notch will be discussed later. Probably a similar significance attaches to the subdivision of the synaptically evoked spike into two components that was reported by Phillips (1956b) for cortical pyramidal cells (Figure 30D) and by Rose and Mountcastle (1954, Figure 2) for thalamic neurones, and to the compound spike potentials recorded by Tasaki, Polley, and Orrego (1954) from lateral geniculate neurones.

4. Stimulation of Motoneurones by Directly Applied Current

As already described, Araki and Otani (1955) were able by a bridge device to apply currents of various durations and intensities through an intracellular microelectrode and to record through the same electrode the intracellular potential so produced in amphibian motoneurones. When an applied current had produced a depolarization of about 9 mV (range 6.5 mV to 11.5 mV), a spike potential was generated which closely resembled that produced by synaptic stimulation. As would be expected from the exponentially increasing depolarization (cf. Figures 6, 7), the latent period for initiation of a spike decreased with increasing intensity of a steady current. With latent periods longer than 7 msec., there was often an increase in the threshold level of depolarization, indicating the onset of accommodation. Frank and Fuortes (1956b) and Coombs, Curtis and Eccles (1956b) have similarly investigated mammalian motoneurones and found that the threshold level of depolarization for initiation of an impulse is about 10 mV.

The application of current through the recording microelectrode, however, has the disadvantage that voltage changes arise within the electrode because of the redistribution of ions. This complication can be avoided by applying the current through one barrel of a double micro-electrode (Figure 3) embedded in a motoneurone, the membrane potential being recorded through the other barrel (cf. Coombs *et al.*, 1955a).

When allowance is made for the voltage drop in the coupling resistance, it can be assumed that the remainder of the recorded potential change is across the motoneu-

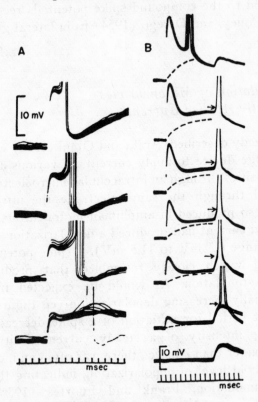

Figure 16

A. Superimposed sweeps displaying membrane potential in a motoneurone on application of rectangular steps of depolarizing current through one barrel of a double microelectrode. Current commences about one-third of the way through each sweep and continues throughout the sweep. Current increases from the bottom to the top record. Both here and in Figure 16B the initial rapid rise of potential and the overshoot of the plateau at the start of the current are artefacts due to capacitative coupling between the two barrels of the microelectrode and are not actually developed across the

ronal membrane. Furthermore, it can be assumed that the surface membrane of the soma, the proximal regions of the dendrites, and the initial segment of the axon are uniformly depolarized by the amount of potential change so calculated. Since the length constant of a standard dendrite has been estimated to be about 300 μ, those parts of the dendritic membrane some hundreds of microns from the soma will be much less depolarized by the applied current. It therefore seems likely that the relationship of depolarization to impulse generation is being studied for the surface membrane of the soma together with the adjacent regions of the large dendrites and the motor axon.

As shown in Figures 16B and 25A, at the onset of the square current pulse there was a capacitative overshoot of the potential, which in the absence of an impulse declined with a time constant of about 1 msec. to a steady level that was maintained indefinitely. This initial capacitative wave prevented the recording of the time course of the membrane depolarization which would be expected to increase exponentially to a plateau with the time course characteristic of the membrane, i.e., with a time constant of about 2.5 msec. The approximate time courses for membrane depolarizations calculated on this basis are indicated in Figure 16B by the broken lines, allowance also being made for the potential developed in the coupling resistance.

Even before these allowances are made, it is seen that

---

cell membrane. Furthermore, about one-sixth of the potential (one-fourth in Figure 16B) making up the plateau is also an artefact due to the resistance coupling of the two barrels and is not developed across the cell membrane. Resting potential was − 64 mV (Coombs, Eccles, and Fatt, 1955a). *B*. Depolarizing currents are applied as in Figure 16A in all but the lowest record, and in addition an afferent volley generates monosynaptically an EPSP toward the end of each sweep. Resting potential was −66 mV. The approximate time courses of the membrane depolarizations produced by the applied currents are indicated by the broken lines (see text). In the uppermost record this depolarization generated an impulse in the motoneurone, while in the remaining records the EPSP was effective by virtue of its superposition on the depolarization, the arrows indicating the approximate potentials at which the spikes were initiated (modified from Coombs, Eccles, and Fatt, 1955a).

a recorded depolarization of less than 10 mV can generate an impulse (Figure 16A). With any one motoneurone, the threshold level of depolarization for a directly applied

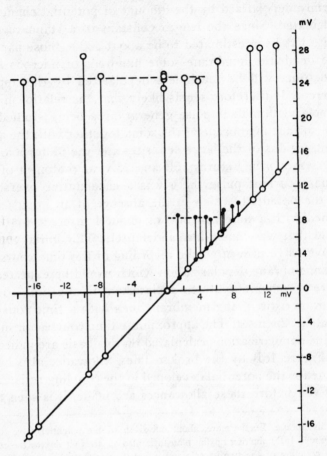

Figure 17

Effect of changes in membrane potential on the generation of impulses in a motoneurone by monosynaptic excitation (filled circles) and by antidromic excitation (open circles). Zero on the abscissal scale is at resting membrane potential (−66 mV), the membrane hyperpolarizations produced by applied current pulses being shown to the left and the depolarizations to the right with due allowance for the potential built up in the coupling resistance. Ordinates also show membrane potential change, so the initial positions produced by the applied pulses before the evoked responses will lie as shown on a 45° line. The vertical lines join these initial positions to the potential at which a spike is initiated. The records giving the filled

current has always been very close to the threshold level of EPSP for the synaptic excitation of an impulse. This suggests that the depolarization of the EPSP has a general causal relationship to the initiation of the impulse discharge, just as occurs with depolarization in giant axons (Cole and Curtis, 1939; Hodgkin, 1948; Hodgkin *et al.*, 1952). This inference can be tested by superimposing a synaptic excitation on a steady depolarizing-current. As shown in Figure 16B, the larger the steady depolarizing potential, the lower is the threshold level of the superimposed synaptic depolarization. In fact, as shown in Figure 17 (horizontal dotted line through filled circles), in the process of generating an impulse, the synaptic depolarization appears to be a very effective substitute for direct depolarization, the two depolarizations being about equipotent in this respect, i.e., the larger the direct depolarization, the smaller is the addition of synaptic depolarization at the instant when the spike arises. It is also of interest that spikes are observed to arise at approximately the same levels of depolarization that are produced by other synaptic mechanisms, e.g., excitation through polysynaptic pathways or by an inhibitory synaptic action that has a depolarizing action because of the high intracellular level of such anions as chloride or nitrate (Figure 40E–G; Figure 41B,C; cf. Coombs *et al.*, 1955b).

EPSP's generated monosynaptically in motoneurones by various sizes of volleys (Figure 10A–C), both in the

---

circles are partly illustrated in Figure 16B, where the arrows signal the origins of the impulses. The vertical lines joining the filled circles in Figure 17 give the respective heights of the EPSP's at these arrows. The records giving the open circles are illustrated in Figure 25A, but much faster recording was used to determine the origins of the SD from the IS spike (cf. Fig. 18) as marked by arrows in Figure 25A. Note that when superimposed on depolarizations up to 7 mV, the EPSP generates a spike at a total depolarization of about 8.4 mV from the resting potential of −66 mV as indicated by the horizontal broken line, while with the antidromic impulse the IS spike has to be at a total depolarization of about 25 mV before the SD spike is generated (upper horizontal broken line). The increased values with larger depolarizing currents are probably due to partial electrode blockage.

afferent nerve of the homonymous muscle and in afferent nerves from synergic muscles, have virtually the same time course. Hence it may be concluded that the synapses activated by these various volleys have no specific regions of distribution. For example, if one type of volley activated synapses on the more remote regions of the dendrites, its EPSP would exhibit the slower time course that arises because of electrotonic transmission, there being in particular a later and more rounded summit. Conversely, preponderant activation of synapses on the soma would result in an EPSP having an earlier and sharper summit followed by a period of decay initially more rapid than exponential. The distortion would be exactly comparable with that observed for the EPP intracellularly recorded at the neuromuscular junction (Fatt and Katz, 1951), where likewise there is distortion because of electrotonic spread of the depolarization to areas of membrane remote from the junctional region. Thus it appears that the monosynaptic excitatory synapses from the various afferent nerves are distributed fairly uniformly over the soma and dendrites of any motoneurone. Hence a microelectrode in the soma will be very favourably placed for recording the mean membrane depolarization produced by a monosynaptic excitatory volley. It would therefore be expected that the synaptically produced depolarization would sum with that directly produced by applied current in causing the generation of impulses, which is precisely in accord with observation (Figures 16B, 17).

Direct stimulation of the motoneurone by applied current further resembles synaptic stimulation in that there is a very brief notch at the same potential level on the rising phase of the spike potential (compare Figure 15C with B; Araki and Otani, 1955; Fatt, 1956b; Coombs, Curtis and Eccles, 1956b). The significance of this important observation will be discussed after an account has been given of the antidromic responses of motoneurones.

5. Stimulation of a Motoneurone by an Impulse Propagating Antidromically up the Motor Axon

The full sequence of potential changes is illustrated in Figure 18A in which current applied through one barrel of

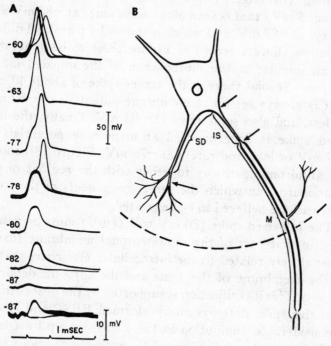

Figure 18

A. Intracellular responses evoked by an antidromic impulse, indicating stages of blockage of the antidromic spike in relation to the initial level of membrane potential. Initial membrane potential (indicated to the left of each record) was controlled by the application of extrinsic currents. Resting potential was at −80 mV. The lowest record was taken after the amplification had been increased 4.5 times and the stimulus had been decreased until it was just at threshold for exciting the axon of the motoneurone (Coombs, Eccles, and Fatt, 1955a). *B.* Schematic drawing of a motoneurone showing dendrites (only one drawn with terminal branches), the soma, the initial segment of axon (IS) and the medullated axon (M) with two nodes, at one of which there is an axon collateral. The three arrows indicate the regions where delay or blockage of an antidromic impulse is likely to occur. The regions producing the M, IS, and SD spikes are indicated approximately by the labelled brackets. (Eccles, 1955).

a double microelectrode changed the membrane potential from the resting level of −80 mV either up as far as −87 mV or down as low as −60 mV. This procedure (Coombs *et al.*, 1955a) shows that the antidromic spike potential has three distinct components, each of all-or-nothing character. There is first the very small spike (about 5 mV) that is seen alone sometimes at −82 mV and always at −87 mV, and which is shown by threshold differentiation (lowest record of Figure 18A) to be generated by an impulse in the motor axon of the impaled motoneurone. Second there is the larger spike of about 40 mV that is always set up at membrane potentials of −80 mV or less, and also sometimes at −82 mV. Finally, the full-sized spike is superimposed at membrane potentials of −77 mV or less, and rarely at −78 mV. Figure 18B shows the antidromic pathway together with the regions of the motoneurone in which the three components of the spike potential are believed to be generated.

The full-sized spike (80 mV to 100 mV) must be generated in that part of the motoneuronal membrane that is most closely related to the intracellular electrode, that is, in the membrane of the soma and the adjacent dendritic regions. This identification is supported by the observations that this spike destroys any preformed EPSP and causes a considerable diminution in the EPSP set up by a later excitatory volley (cf. Figure 12). Such observations indicate that the full-sized spike has invaded those regions of the surface membrane on which the synaptic knobs are concentrated and which are shown histologically to be the soma and the adjacent dendritic regions. The full-sized spike may therefore be termed the soma-dendritic, or SD, spike (Brock, Coombs, and Eccles, 1953; J. C. Eccles, 1955).

The spike of 30 mV to 40 mV has been ascribed to the nonmedullated axon and axon hillock, and has been termed the NM spike (Brock *et al.*, 1952a; 1953; Woodbury and Patton, 1952; J. C. Eccles, 1955; Araki and Otani, 1955; Frank and Fuortes, 1955b), but it is now proposed to utilize the more convenient collective term "initial segment" for these two components and the consequent abbreviation "IS spike." This identification of the origin of the IS spike has been based on the likelihood of a block in antidromic transmission at the axon hillock, where there is such a large expansion in the surface membrane to be invaded. It will later emerge that antidromic blockage at this site is aided greatly by the much higher threshold of the soma-dendritic membrane. The identification is supported further by the observation that, provided no SD spike is generated, the IS spike and the EPSP are virtually additive in the depolarization recorded by a microelectrode in the soma (Brock, Coombs, and Eccles, 1953; Fatt, 1956b; Coombs, Curtis and Eccles, 1956b), which indicates that the IS spike arises in a part of the motoneurone on which there are few, if any, excitatory synapses, i.e., in the motor axon. On the other hand, the relatively large size of the IS spike indicates that it arises in an area of membrane very close to the soma and even encroaching on it. Thus, as indicated in Figure 18B, it is proposed that the IS spike arises from the axon hillock as well as the nonmedullated axon, i.e., from the initial segment of the axon.

Finally the very small spike (1 mV to 5 mV) has been ascribed to the medullated axon and has been termed the M spike (Brock, Coombs, and Eccles, 1953; J. C. Eccles, 1955). This identification has been based on its small size and the likelihood of blockage when the impulse in the medullated axon, where only the very small nodal areas are activated, attempts to invade the large surface area of the initial segment of the axon. It is supported by its all-or-nothing character, by the short refractory period that follows the M spike, and by its ability to follow high frequencies of stimulation. In all these respects it resembles spikes in medullated axons.

Systematic surveys of the extracellular potential fields generated by the motoneurones of a motor nucleus (Lorente de Nó, 1947; 1953; Lloyd, 1951a) and more recently by a single motoneurone (Fatt, 1956a) have shown that an antidromic impulse propagates very slowly along the dendrites, the mean velocity being as low as 2 metres a sec. and even as low as 0.7 metres a sec. in the more remote regions. The potential fields further indicate that there may be blockage of the antidromic impulse before it has invaded the extreme dendritic terminals (Barakan, Downman, and Eccles, 1949; J. C. Eccles, 1950), a possibility first suggested by Toennies and Jung (1948) and further developed by Jung (1953a). On the local-circuit theory of impulse propagation this progressive slowing and eventual blockage is to be expected because the dendrites become progressively more tenuous (cf. Lorente de Nó, 1953; Chu, 1954), so increasing the ratio of surface capacitance to core conductance, and this ratio is increased further by the profuse branching (cf. Barakan *et al.*, 1949).

6. *Discussion on Sites of Origin of Impulses*

If the above identification of sites of the three kinds of antidromic spike potentials is well founded, it should be possible to give satisfactory explanations of the spike potentials generated synaptically and by the directly applied current. Since the notch on the rising phases of both these kinds of spike potentials is always at the same potential as the origin of the SD spike from the IS spike during antidromic invasion, e.g., all occur at about 30 mV depolarization in Figure 15 (cf. Araki and Otani, 1955; Frank and Fuortes, 1956b; Fatt, 1956b; Coombs, Curtis, and Eccles, 1956b), it can be concluded that with synaptic and direct stimulation an IS spike also precedes an SD spike. Thus, in all three cases it is envisaged (cf. Araki and Otani, 1955) that the invasion of the soma-dendritic membrane is preceded by a spike in the initial segment (Figure 15). The threshold of 6 mV to 15 mV that has been measured for both synaptic and direct stimulation (Figures 14, 15B, 16, 24, 41H) is therefore the threshold for generating an impulse (IS impulse) in the initial segment. Approximately three times that depolarization (i.e., 20 mV to 40 mV) is required to generate a spike in the soma-dendritic membrane (cf. Figures 14, 15, 18, 19). It is given by the IS spike, plus the value of the field potential (about 1 mV) that is recorded simultaneously and in the opposite direction by an extracellular electrode (Fatt, 1956a). Figures 17 (open circles) and 25A show that, in the generation of an SD spike, potential changes produced by current pulses sum directly with the depolarization produced by the IS spike. For example, over a wide range of initial membrane potentials, the open circles in Figure 17 lie along the horizontal broken line at 25.5 mV depolarization. The situation resembles precisely that for the generation of the IS spike (filled circles in Figure 17) except that the threshold depolarization is three times greater.

By recording the potential fields around a single motoneurone that is being invaded antidromically, Fatt (1956a) has shown that during the IS spike, as would be expected, large currents flow into the motoneurone (apparently into the initial segment) while the soma-dendritic membrane is being depolarized by the threshold amount of approximately 30 mV. When the impulse then invades the soma-dendritic membrane, there is a still larger inward current as the more remote dendritic regions are being progressively depolarized.

The above solution to the problem of spike origins removes one anomaly that has been difficult to explain—the much higher threshold that appeared to obtain for antidromic invasion of the soma-dendritic membrane (30 mV as against 10 mV for synaptic and direct stimulation). There is substituted, however, the difficulty of explaining why the threshold of the soma-dendritic membrane is three times as high as that of the initial segment.

A possible suggestion could be that the soma-dendritic membrane has a high threshold because it is so densely covered by synaptic knobs and even by glial cells (Wyckoff and Young, 1956), whereas there are relatively few synapses on the initial segment (Hoff, 1932a; Lorente de Nó, 1938; Barr, 1939). On analogy with the subsynaptic membrane of the neuromuscular junction, i.e., the end-plate membrane (Fatt and Katz, 1951), with the whole membrane of the slow fibres of amphibian muscles (Kuffler and Vaughan Williams, 1953; Burke and Ginsborg, 1955), and with the modified junctional material of the electric organs of Torpedo (Fessard, 1946; 1952; Fessard and Posternak, 1950; Albe-Fessard, 1951) and of the ray (Brock, Eccles, and Keynes, 1953), it is possible that the subsynaptic areas of membrane are incapable of responding by impulses. Such areas may form at least 50 per cent of the total soma membrane, and would act to shunt any regenerative depolarization, i.e., incipient impulses, in the remainder of the membrane. Only a small increase in threshold could be explained in this way, so it would seem that either glial coverage or some intrinsic difference in the membrane, or both together, must also be invoked if a three fold increase in threshold is to be explained. An intrinsic difference in the membrane is suggested by cytological evidence which distinguishes between the soma and the initial segment (Chang, 1952; Chu, 1954), and is strongly indicated by the after-potentials, the after-hyperpolarization being large after the SD spike and undetectable after the IS spike (Coombs et al., 1955a).

It must be assumed that, when an IS spike fails to invade the soma-dendritic membrane, this membrane is depolarized almost by the amount of that spike, about 30 mV, and yet rapid repolarization ensues on its termination (cf. Figure 18A at -80 mV and -82 mV), which contrasts with the relatively slow exponential decay after an EPSP. In part, this difference arises because the decay of the EPSP is slowed by the residual subsynaptic current (cf. Figure 11A), but the initial decline of the IS spike is much more rapid than can be accounted for by a membrane time constant of about 2.5 msec. A possible explanation (cf. Brock, Coombs, and Eccles, 1953) is that during the decline of the IS spike a current that repolarizes th soma is generated by the high K⁺ conductance of the areas that were producing the currents giving the IS spike, i.e., by the initial segment. On the contrary, with amphibian motoneurones, the IS spike has a much slower repolarization (Araki *et al.*, 1953), which is also observed with the crustacean stretch receptor cells (cf. Figure 33C; Eyzaguirre and Kuffler, 1955b). Presumably in these situations the polarizing current from the axon is much less effective.

The IS-SD interval for synaptic and direct stimulation would be expected to be much shorter than for antidromic invasion because the SD membrane is already depolarized before the IS spike is generated (Coombs, Curtis and Eccles, 1956b; Frank and Fuortes, 1956b). If the IS-SD interval is measured between the origins of the respective spikes, especially as shown in the electrically differentiated records, it is 0.25 msec. to 0.5 msec. for antidromic impulses (Figures 14G, 15A, 18A) and usually less than 0.2 msec. for spikes evoked by direct or synaptic stimulation (Figures 14B–F; 15B,C). A similar brief IS-SD interval is observed when antidromic invasion occurs into an SD membrane already depolarized by an EPSP or by a directly applied current (Figure 18A at −63 mV; cf. Araki and Otani, 1955).

The same explanation accounts for the difficulty in producing an IS-SD blockage in a normal motoneurone that is stimulated directly or synaptically. Any attempt to raise the threshold for an SD spike, as for example by hyperpolarizing the membrane or by a preliminary antidromic invasion, also raises the threshold for generating the IS spike. Since the IS spike then arises from a stronger synaptic or direct stimulus, the increased preliminary depolarization will likewise aid the IS-SD invasion. However, a considerable lengthening of the IS-SD interval can be produced by this procedure, as may be seen in the responses of Figure 19C,D at a test interval just critical for blockage of all the spike responses (cf. Figure 19B,E). The later responses to a repetitive train of presynaptic volleys also exhibit lengthening of the IS-SD interval, and even

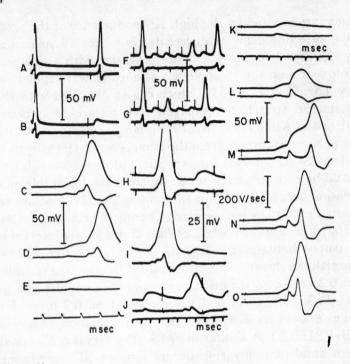

Figure 19

A–E. Effect of a preceding antidromic volley on the generation of a spike by monosynaptic excitation. At an interval of 22 msec., recovery of excitability has attained a critical stage at which an EPSP sometimes generates a spike, *A*, or fails, *B*. Faster recording shows finer details of the spike in *C* and *D*, and of the EPSP alone in *E*. Beneath each potential record there is an electrically differentiated record, which shows in *C* and *D* an IS-SD interval of about 0.35 msec. *F–J.* Same motoneurone as in *A–E*, but responding to brief repetitive presynaptic volleys at about 230 a sec. Note that in *F* the fifth and in *G* the third responses have a small spike superimposed on the EPSP's. Detailed analysis is shown in *H–J*, with the subjacent electrically differentiated records, which show respectively the first two, the last two, and two intermediate responses of the repetitive series. The tops of the large spikes are truncated, but the IS-SD separation is considerable in *I*, while in *J* the second response is clearly an IS spike superimposed on an EPSP. *K–O*. A series of responses evoked in another motoneurone by a monosynaptic volley, there being also electrically differentiated records below the potential responses. This motoneurone was in a deteriorated condition. A maximum volley evoked a spike with a large IS-SD separation, *O*, while with progressive weakening of the volley the IS-SD interval increased (*N–M*) and in *L* the SD spike failed. With still further weakening the IS spike also failed, leaving only the EPSP (*K*). (Coombs, Curtis, and Eccles, 1956b).

blockage, with only IS spikes arising from the EPSP (Figure 19G,J). Such responses are exhibited especially by deteriorated motoneurones, and Figure 19 K–O shows lengthening of the IS-SD interval (up to 1.5 msec. in M) and the simple IS spike (L) that may be produced under such conditions by a single presynaptic volley when its size is reduced so that the EPSP is just at threshold for generating a spike (cf. Coombs *et al.*, 1955c, p. 382).

Many years ago Forbes (1934, 1939), Gesell (1940), and more recently P. O. Bishop (1953) put forward an hypothesis identical with that proposed here and by Araki and Otani (1955), i.e., that the synaptically evoked impulses arise at the initial segment. Crucial evidence on such detailed behaviour of a neurone, however, could be derived only by intracellular recording. It is of interest that the especially low threshold (about 10 mV depolarization) of the initial segment makes much more effective use of the depolarizing and hyperpolarizing currents that are generated by synaptic excitatory and inhibitory action respectively. Furthermore, far better integration of the whole synaptic excitatory and inhibitory bombardment is provided by this arrangement than by the impulses being generated anywhere over the whole soma-dendritic membrane. If these latter conditions obtained, a special strategic grouping of excitatory synapses (cf. Lorente de Nó, 1938) could initiate an impulse despite a relative paucity of the total excitatory synaptic bombardment and a considerable inhibitory bombardment of areas remote from this focus. Such a breakdown of the integrative function of a motoneurone is prevented by the high threshold of the soma-dendritic membrane relative to the initial segment. Since synapses can thus be effective only in so far as they can depolarize the initial segment, those synapses remotely placed on dendrites will be functionally ineffective in view of the estimated space constant of 300 μ. Possibly this relative ineffectiveness may be correlated with the sparse distribution in such regions (Lorente de Nó, 1938; Barr, 1939; Bodian, 1952). It should be noted that the origin of the spike in the initial segment may be a special feature of motoneurones. It cannot be demonstrated with sympathetic ganglion cells (Figure 31J), and impulses can be generated in the apical dendrites of pyramidal cells (Cragg and Hamlyn, 1955).

7. The Current That Flows during the EPSP

It has been shown (cf. Figure 11) that brief depolarizing currents are responsible for the EPSP, which is a depolarization of the soma-dendritic and axonal membranes. In order to produce this effect the currents must be flowing in an outward direction across these postsynaptic membranes and there must be a corresponding inward current across the subsynaptic membranes of the activated synapses (Figure 11B). More detailed consideration of the flow of this inward current in relationship to the synaptic knobs will be attempted later. Our present problems concern the voltage that causes this postsynaptic current flow and the ionic mechanisms that are responsible for it.

Experimental evidence relating to the voltage can be obtained by varying the membrane potential of the motoneurone by passing a steady current through one barrel of a double microelectrode while the EPSP is recorded as a superimposed transient change by means of the other barrel (cf. Figure 20). The membrane potential for each record of Figure 20 is calculated by subtracting from the observed steady potential the potential that the applied current would generate in the coupling resistance (cf. Figure 4). For example, if a steady current of 5×10^{-8}A diminished the intracellularly recorded potential from -70 mV to -10 mV, and the coupling resistance as measured extracellularly was $200,000\Omega$, 10 mV of the change would arise in the coupling resistance and the actual membrane potential would have been diminished only to -20 mV. Under such conditions the applied depolarizing current would have caused repetitive discharge of impulses by the

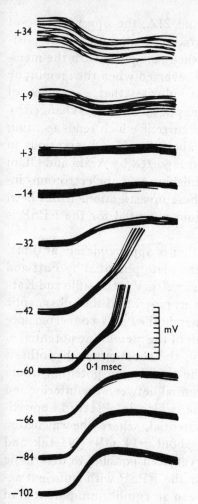

+34

+9

+3

−14

−32

−42

mV

0.1 msec

−60

−66

−84

−102

Figure 20

EPSP's set up in a biceps-semitendinosus motoneurone at various levels of membrane potential. Membrane potentials are indicated in mV to the left of each record as the potential of the interior of the cell with respect to the exterior. The resting potential was at −66 mV; the other potentials were obtained by the application of an extrinsic current through one barrel of a double microelectrode. In each record decreasing internal negativity (depolarization from the resting level) or increasing internal positivity is upward. The records are each formed by superimposing 15 to 20 sweeps with the response occurring at the same relative time during the sweep. The scatter of individual sweeps in the records at greatest internal positivity is caused by fluctuations in the initial level of membrane potential. Spike potentials are evoked by the EPSP at membrane potentials of −42 mV and −60 mV (Coombs, Eccles, and Fatt, 1955c).

motoneurone. Usually this discharge ceased in a few seconds and the observations on the EPSP could then be made. If the microelectrode was filled with a potassium salt, it was found that, on cessation of such a depolarizing current, all responses of the motoneurone recovered within a few seconds to the initial conditions obtaining before the application of the current. It may therefore be assumed that the current had no deleterious effect on the motoneurone.

As shown in Figures 20 and 21A, the upward slope of the EPSP, which is an approximate measure of the post-synaptic current, was diminished *pari passu* with the membrane potential, and actually reversed when the membrane potential was reversed. This indicates that, regardless of its initial potential, the subsynaptic membrane is changed by activation so that it passes a current which tends to bring the membrane potential to about 0 mV. Observations in general agreement have been reported by Araki and Otani (1955), catelectrotonus diminishing and anelectrotonus increasing the EPSP. From these investigations it has been concluded that the equilibrium potential for the EPSP is approximately at 0 mV.

An equilibrium potential that is approximately at 0 mV has been observed for the end plate potential by Fatt and Katz (1951) and at −10 mV to −20 mV by Castillo and Katz (1954e). They consequently proposed that the subsynaptic membrane (the end-plate membrane) was converted momentarily to be a short-circuit of the membrane potential of the muscle fibre. Actually on the short-circuit hypothesis it would be expected that the equilibrium potential would be at the liquid-junction potential between the interior and exterior of the motoneurone, which is observed approximately for the end-plate potential, where the calculated liquid-junction potential is about −14 mV (Nastuk and Hodgkin, 1950). It has not yet been possible to determine the equilibrium potential for the EPSP with sufficient accuracy to discriminate between an equilibrium potential of 0 mV and such an assumed liquid-junction potential.

If the subsynaptic membrane is converted by the transmitter substance into a short-circuit, it would be expected that it would be equally permeable to all ions. This inference can be tested by changing the ionic composition of the motoneurone by injecting ions electrophoretically through the microelectrode. By this means large changes can be produced in the other electrical responses of the motoneurone, the membrane potential, the spike potential, the after-hyperpolarization following a spike, and the in-

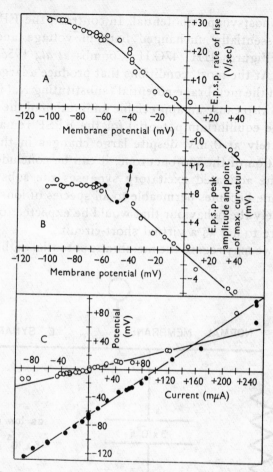

Figure 21

A. Plotting of maximum rate of rise of EPSP against initial level of membrane potential for series partly shown in Figure 20. Ordinates are the time rates of decreasing internal negativity (or increasing internal positivity); abscissae are potentials of interior of motoneurone with respect to exterior. *B.* Plot of peak amplitude of EPSP (open circles) and point of maximum curvature at start of action potential (filled circles) against initial level of membrane potential. Ordinates are amplitudes of transient decrease of internal negativity (or increase of internal positivity) produced by the EPSP; abscissae as in *A.* *C.* Plot of steady level of potential recorded inside the motoneurone (filled circles) and after withdrawing from the motoneurone (open circles) against applied current. Ordinates are potentials at orifice of microelectrode with respect to distant surroundings; abscissae are currents applied by microelectrode, the direction outward from the orifice being positive (Coombs, Eccles, and Fatt, 1955c).

hibitory postsynaptic potential. In contrast, the EPSP remains essentially unchanged both in voltage and time course (Figures 41H; 47G,H; Coombs *et al.*, 1955c, Figure 10). At the most, conditions that produce a large diminution of the membrane potential (substituting Na^+ ions for K^+ ions) also cause an appreciable diminution of the EPSP. Since the equilibrium potential for the EPSP remains approximately at 0 mV despite large changes in the ionic composition of the motoneurone, it can be concluded that under the activated excitatory synapses the subsynaptic membrane becomes permeable to all species of ions, which is precisely the behaviour that would be expected to obtain if it were to act as a virtual short-circuit.

Thus we may regard the membrane potential of the soma-

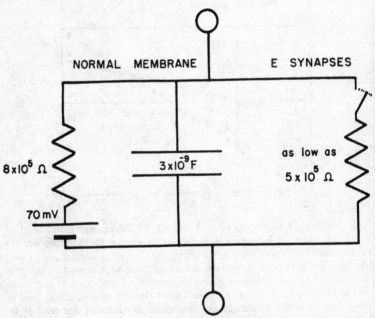

Figure 22

Formal electrical diagram of the membrane of a motoneurone (cf. Figure 9) with, on the right side, the circuit through the subsynaptic areas of the membrane that are activated in producing the monosynaptic EPSP. Maximum activation of these areas would be indicated symbolically by closing the switch.

dendritic and adjacent axonal regions as providing the voltage that causes the excitatory postsynaptic current to flow inward through the subsynaptic membrane under the activated excitatory synaptic knobs (cf. Figure 11B). If the equilibrium potential for the EPSP is at 0 mV, the generation of the EPSP can be shown in the formal electrical diagram of Figure 22, wherein are inserted the values determined for the standard motoneurone (Figure 9). The monosynaptic excitatory synapses are shown by a switch in series with a resistance of $5 \times 10^5 \Omega$, which approximately represents the lowest short-circuiting resistance that we have observed. The steepest slope of the EPSP was about 50V per sec., which would require a current of 15×10^{-8}A to discharge the membrane capacity of 3×10^{-9}F. This current would be produced if a potential of 70 mV were connected through a short-circuiting resistance of about $5 \times 10^5 \Omega$. Actually this resistance is produced by a large number of much higher resistances in parallel. Perhaps as many as several hundred activated excitatory synapses are required to produce an EPSP with a slope of 50V per sec.

In Figure 20 hyperpolarization of the membrane to −84 mV caused the EPSP to rise more steeply to an earlier summit, effects which were accentuated at −102 mV. Figure 23C shows typically that the time course of decay is also accelerated by a hyperpolarization of 30 mV, the time constant of 4.6 msec. in Figure 23B being shortened to 3.0 msec. According to the short-circuit hypothesis, it would be expected that the intensity of the subsynaptic current (the current plotted in Figure 11A), and hence the rising slope of the EPSP, would be proportional to the membrane potential. As we have seen, this relationship approximately obtains for the depolarizing range (below −66 mV in Figure 21A), but on the other hand with hyperpolarization the slope increases much more slowly. The diminishing effectiveness of hyperpolarization is more evident if the summit of the EPSP is plotted instead of the maximum slope, for usually there is no significant change

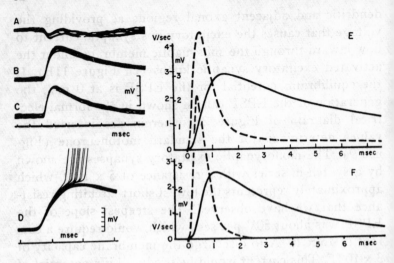

Figure 23

A, B, and C are monosynaptic EPSP's of a gastrocnemius motoneurone, B being at the resting potential (about −70 mV) while with C the membrane was hyperpolarized by about 30 mV and with A, depolarized so that the level of membrane potential was reversed by about 10 mV. D. Responses in a different motoneurone from that illustrated in A–C, showing the mode of origin of spikes from an EPSP of critical amplitude. The rapid upstroke of the spikes has been retouched to restore losses in photography. The membrane potential was initially at its resting level (−74 mV) (Coombs, Eccles, and Fatt, 1955c). E, F. The time courses of the subsynaptic currents generating the EPSP's of the B and C responses (continuous lines) have been calculated as in Figure 11A and plotted as broken lines, the scales in V/sec. being convertible into current scales as in Figure 11A. Note that for economy of plotting, the curve for F is drawn overlapping the curves for E. The time constant of the membrane was not directly determined, but was assumed to be 2.8 msec., which on the basis of other experiments may be chosen as a reasonable value for an EPSP that decays with a time constant of 4.6 msec. at the resting membrane potential (Figure 23 B).

for a wide range of hyperpolarization, as is shown by the open circles from −66 mV to −102 mV in Figure 21B.

No satisfactory explanation has been developed hitherto for the wide deviation from a linear relationship between the hyperpolarized membrane potentials and the EPSP's (cf. Coombs *et al.*, 1955c). The considerable shortening that hyperpolarization produces in the time constant of decay of the EPSP (Figure 23B–C) also has been inexplicable, because simultaneous measurements showed that there was no appreciable diminution in membrane resistance (Figure 21C; cf. Coombs *et al.*, 1955c). It seems that these difficulties and inconsistencies can be resolved satisfactorily, now that the time constant of decay of the EPSP is recognized as being compounded of a briefer membrane time-constant (about 2.5 msec.) and a decaying residuum of subsynaptic current (cf. broken line of Figure 11A). Since the measured membrane resistance is constant over the hyperpolarizing range (cf. filled circles of Figure 21C), it is justifiable to assume that the time-constant of the membrane is unchanged; hence the alteration in the EPSP must be effected by a change in the time course of the subsynaptic current, as is illustrated by the calculated curves of Figure 23 E–F. Not only does this current decay much more rapidly, but also its initial summit is less than would be expected for a linear relationship to membrane potential. Thus, the hyperpolarizing current has been interfering either with the process whereby transmitter substance is removed from the proximity of the subsynaptic membrane, or with the actual attachment of the transmitter substance to the subsynaptic membrane, i.e., by a curare-like action. The former postulate is more attractive because of its simplicity, for, if the transmitter substance is negatively charged, it would be carried away from the subsynaptic membrane by the hyperpolarizing current that penetrates it. This postulate accounts for the relative deficiency in the initial summit as well as for the greatly increased rate of decay of the subsynaptic current in Figure 23F.

This simple postulate also can contribute to the explanation of the diminished size, the earlier summit and the faster decay of the EPSP that is set up during the hyperpolarization following a spike potential (cf. Figure 12B). If the hyperpolarization is generated only by that part of the postsynaptic membrane invaded by the spike and hence probably unrelated to synapses (as suggested above), it will cause an inward current to flow through the sub-synaptic areas of the membrane, which in effect will be the same as an extrinsically applied hyperpolarizing current. Finally, the postulate may explain also the initial very rapid decline of the subsynaptic current (cf. Figures 11A, 23E), for this current will be flowing across the subsynaptic membrane in the same direction as an extrinsic hyperpolarizing current (cf. Figure 11B) and will be of much greater intensity; hence it should cause a very rapid removal of a transmitter substance that is negatively charged. The residual current in Figures 11A and 23E would be due to the continued action of the small amount of transmitter substance that survived this rapid removal by electric current.

8. Discussion on the Initiation of Impulses

Since intracellular recording from motoneurones has shown that the generation of impulses by monosynaptic excitation is satisfactorily accountable to the depolarization of the initial segment which is produced by the ionic currents across the membrane, i.e., to the EPSP, it is necessary to examine the evidence which has been regarded as being incompatible with this explanation. This evidence has been derived from a precise analysis of the relation between the size of an afferent volley and its effectiveness in evoking reflex discharges from one motoneurone or from assemblages of motoneurones (Lloyd and McIntyre, 1955; Hunt, 1955). The effectiveness of the test volleys was varied by means of post-tetanic potentiation and by synaptic facilitatory action. Essentially this evidence has shown that the "transmitter potentiality" of an impulse decays considerably in 0.2 msec. to 0.3 msec., which is in contrast with the much longer duration of the EPSP. The comparison, however, should have been made with the time course of the ionic current across the subsynaptic membrane, because impulses are generated only during the phase of incrementing depolarization produced by these currents. There is no incompatibility between the time course of the current in Figures 11A and 23E (broken lines) and a transmitter potentiality that decays considerably in 0.2 msec. to 0.3 msec.

The problem of relating membrane depolarization to impulse generation is illustrated further in Figure 23D, where the strength of stimulus applied to the afferent nerve was just at the threshold for evoking a reflex discharge from the impaled motoneurone. In about half of the series of over 20 superimposed responses it is seen that a spike potential was generated and that it arose relatively late in the rising phase of the EPSP. Close examination shows that, relative to the EPSP recorded in the absence of a spike potential, a slow upward creep of potential always preceded the sharp upward deflection of the spike itself. With motoneurones in good physiological condition deviation between the two classes of records occurs about 0.5 msec. before the EPSP attains its summit (Coombs *et al.*, 1955c). The slow increase in depolarization beyond this point is not able to initiate the discharge of an impulse. The process giving rise to an impulse in the initial segment either has been initiated at least 0.5 msec. earlier than the summit or it fails altogether.

The ineffectiveness of the terminal slowly-rising phase of the EPSP probably is an example of accommodation of the initial segment. The direct application of a steady depolarizing current gives further evidence of this accommodation. When sufficiently large (1 to 2 x 10^{-8}A), such currents evoke a repetitive discharge of impulses, but the frequency declines progressively, and the discharge often ceases in a few seconds. Presumably this accommodative process resembles that observed in giant axons (Hodgkin, 1948; Hodgkin and Huxley, 1952c), and may be similarly explained. This accommodation of the impulse-generating mechanism during a steady depolarization, however, makes it difficult to explain the steady frequency of discharge which can be evoked by a prolonged uniform synaptic bombardment (Adrian and Bronk, 1929; Denny-Brown, 1929; Alvord and Fuortes, 1953). Possibly accommodation is not effective under such conditions because the depolarization is not uniformly maintained but rather exhibits the unsteadiness which would be expected to arise because of its generation and maintenance by random synaptic bombardment. Presumably such random synaptic bombardment occurs with motoneurones of unanesthetized preparations and may account for the steady frequency or very slow decline of discharge which has been observed in response to a prolonged depolarizing current (Barron and Matthews, 1938; Alanis, 1953; Fuortes, 1954). In a few experiments with motoneurones exhibiting an intense synaptic noise (cf. Brock *et al.*, 1952a), it has been found that the repetitive discharge evoked by a depolarizing current continued throughout the whole duration of currents that flowed for many minutes (Coombs, Curtis, and Eccles, 1956b).

9. *The EPSP and Temporal Facilitation*

If spatial facilitation is inadequate, the excitatory action of a synapse may fail to generate an impulse; nevertheless, it is not ineffective. The relatively enduring EPSP is of importance in giving temporal facilitation of later synaptic excitatory actions. For example, in Figure 24 an afferent volley was unable to generate an impulse either alone or at an interval of 5 or more msec. after a preceding volley. With successive shortening of the test interval, an impulse was generated and its latency was progressively diminished. At such intervals the response to the second volley appears to have been facilitated by the residual depolarization of the EPSP generated by the first volley. A similar facilitatory effect is observed when the depolarization is produced by the application of an extrinsic current through one barrel of a double microelectrode. For example, in Figure 20 the afferent volley failed to generate an impulse

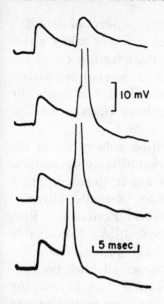

10 mV

5 msec

Figure 24

Intracellular potentials set up in a biceps-semitendinosus motoneurone by two afferent volleys in the biceps-semitendinosus nerve. The volley interval is progressively decreased from above downward. Note the generation of a spike potential (truncated) at all but the longest volley interval. The latency of the spike decreases as the interval shortens.

at the resting potential (-66 mV), but was invariably successful when there was a depolarization of 6 mV (at -60 mV) or 24 mV (at -42 mV).

Further evidence correlating this facilitating influence with the EPSP is provided when the time course of the facilitation is determined by statistical sampling of the monosynaptic reflex discharges from a pool of motoneurones. When the conditioning afferent volley is in a different nerve, the facilitation of the reflex response produced by the test afferent volley diminishes exponentially with lengthening of the test interval, the time constant of decay being about 4 msec. (Lloyd, 1946). It seems likely that the observed reaction of accommodation would account for the small discrepancy between this value and the mean time constant of decay (4.7 msec.) observed for the EPSP. A decay with a time constant of about 4 msec. is also observed for the facilitation which the EPSP exerts on the antidromic invasion of motoneurone somas (Brooks and Eccles, 1947b).

Thus the temporal facilitation of synaptic excitatory actions is explained satisfactorily by the depolarization of the EPSP. When superimposed upon a level of depolarization above a critical value, the test afferent volley is able to initiate an impulse. The lower the effectiveness of the testing volley, the higher is the critical level of depolarization upon which it must be superimposed, and hence the shorter the range of testing intervals at which facilitation is observed.

When the conditioning and testing volleys are in the same afferent fibres, the initial period of temporal facilitation passes over at an interval of about 10 msec. into a depression which persists for many seconds (Brooks, Downman, and Eccles, 1950b; Brock, Eccles, and Rall, 1951; Eccles and Rall, 1951b; Lloyd, 1956). Presumably this prolonged depression is attributable to some change in the presynaptic fibres, for it is not observed when the testing volley is in a different group of afferent fibres from the conditioning, though still exciting the same motoneurones monosynaptically. Under such conditions, however, a small and much briefer depressed phase also occurs after the initial period of facilitation—from about 15 msec. to 100 msec. (Brooks *et al.*, 1950b; Fuortes, 1954). A satisfactory explanation of this relatively brief depression is provided by the small hyperpolarization which has been observed to follow the EPSP (Figure 10D,E).

10. The Spike Potential

a. Time course and voltage

It has already been shown that the full-sized spike potential of 80 mV to 100 mV is composed of an initial IS spike of 30 mV to 40 mV on which the large SD spike is superimposed after a brief interval, which is 0.2 msec. to 0.5 msec. for an antidromically initiated spike and less than 0.2 msec. for spikes initiated by synaptic and direct stimulation. The total duration of the IS-SD spike potential of motoneurones in good condition has never been in our experience longer than 1.5 msec. (cf. Figures 14, 15, 18) and it may be less than 1 msec. (Brock *et al.*, 1952a, Table 1). The observations of Frank and Fuortes (1955b) appear to be in agreement, because the frequently observed durations in excess of 1.5 msec. were probably given by deteriorated motoneurones. A duration of 1.0 msec. was reported by Woodbury and Patton (1952). The heights of the spikes would be reduced by about 20 per cent by the capacity in our recording system, the SD spike being actually about 110 mV (cf. Brock *et al.*, 1952a; Frank and Fuortes, 1955b). With badly injured neurones, however, the spike potentials were of lower voltage, irregular form, and longer duration (cf. Figure 19 L–O), features which are attributable to the irregular and slow propagation of the impulse from the initial segment into the soma and thence along the dendrites. Furthermore, under such conditions, when the excitatory process is just inadequate for generating an impulse, it often sets up a small spike-like process or local response (cf. lowest record, Figure 16A). Hence, in general, the responses of neurones closely resemble those of giant axons.

When the membrane potential is altered by the application of current through one barrel of a double microelectrode, the spike potential shows a corresponding alteration (Figures 4, 25A), which is approximately compensatory except with large depolarizations, i.e., the membrane potential at the spike peak attains almost the same value regardless of the level at which the membrane potential has been set initially (Figures 4, 25B). With large depolarizations the spike potential is reduced more than is necessary for compensation. With amphibian motoneurones Araki and Otani (1955) have observed a less effective compensation.

As described above, it is possible to alter the ionic composition of a motoneurone by passing a current through a microelectrode filled with an appropriate salt. For example, if a current is passed into a motoneurone through a microelectrode filled with a concentrated sodium salt, it is largely carried into the neurone by Na^+ ions and leaves

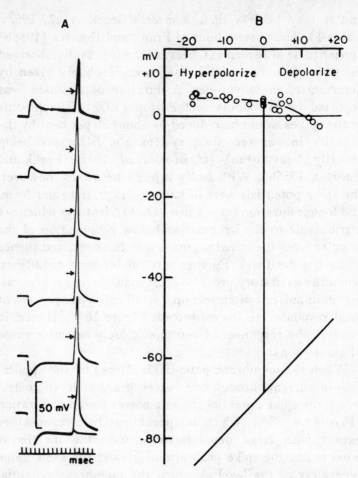

Figure 25

A. Electrical potentials recorded through one barrel of a double micro-electrode when rectangular current pulses are applied through the other barrel as in Figure 16. The pulses begin near the onset of the trace and an antidromic impulse is set up toward the end. For each current the potential level at which the antidromic IS spike generates the SD spike was determined on faster records (not shown) and is indicated in *A* by the arrows. *B.* Plotting of series partly shown in Figure 25A, and largely according to the convention adopted for Figure 17. The changes which the applied currents produce in the membrane potential are plotted as abscissae, allowance being made for the potential produced in the coupling resistance. Zero is resting membrane potential. Zero on ordinate scale indicates zero potential across the moto-neuronal membrane. The plotted points give the membrane potentials at the summits of the spike potentials. There is a reversal of about 5 mV at the

across the surface membrane of the neurone mainly by the outward passage of K^+ ions. In Figure 26A the current of $4 \times 10^{-8}A$ for 120 seconds will have added about 25 p. equiv. of Na^+ to the cell and depleted its potassium by about 20 p. equiv. Since a standard motoneurone contains about 35 p. equiv. of K^+ ions, at least half will have been removed when the current ceased.

It is seen typically in Figure 26A that immediately after the passage of this current an antidromic impulse in the motor axon failed to invade the soma and dendrites of the neurone. There was merely an IS spike which was diminished in size and had an abnormally long time course. Invasion was first observed after about 20 sec., but the spike potential was then small and very prolonged. Thereafter progressive recovery occurred, so that a normal spike potential was observed about 300 sec. later.

Significant changes in the spike potential were also observed when tetramethylammonium or choline ions were injected. Under such conditions, however, the most prominent change was a slowing of the falling phase of the spike (Figure 27 E–F), an effect which was particularly large after a choline injection, and recovery was at best incomplete (Coombs *et al.*, 1955a). The slower rise of the SD spike is attributable largely to the diminution that is produced in the membrane potential. The injection of a wide variety of anions caused little change in the spike potential, any effect being apparently secondary to the small diminution of membrane potential.

All of the experimental observations on the neuronal spike potential are explained satisfactorily by the hypothesis that the spike potential arises because of a brief high permeability, first to Na^+ ions, and then to K^+ ions (Hodgkin and Katz, 1949; Hodgkin, 1951; Hodgkin and

normal membrane potential and with hyperpolarization therefrom. Line at 45° plots the initial membrane potentials from which the spikes arose, the vertical line at 0 giving the spike height at the normal membrane potential (about -74 mV). With large depolarizations the diminution of the spike potential was larger than the change in membrane potential.

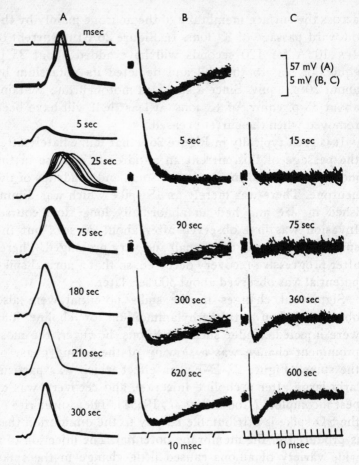

A   **B**   **C**

msec

57 mV (A)
5 mV (B, C)

5 sec

5 sec   15 sec

25 sec

90 sec   75 sec

75 sec

180 sec

300 sec   360 sec

210 sec

620 sec   600 sec

300 sec

10 msec   10 msec

Figure 26

Effect of the injection of Na⁺ ions on the antidromic spike and after-hyperpolarization of a motoneurone, the microelectrode being filled with Na_2SO_4 (1.2 equiv. per litre). After obtaining the top record in *A*, the Na⁺ content of the motoneurone was increased by about 25 p. equiv. by applying a depolarizing current of 4×10^{-8}A for 120 sec., and the further records in A were obtained at the approximate times indicated following the injection. Complete recovery had occurred by the time of the last record in *A*, and the top record of *B* was then taken. This was followed by the injection of approx. 35 p. equiv. Na⁺ (applying 5×10^{-8}A for 150 sec.) and the remaining records in *B* and *C* were taken at the indicated times after the injection. All records are formed by superposition of about forty faint traces. In *A* the resting potential was the same at 5 sec. after the injection as before, although it is probable that the resting potential was not steady by the time of the first record, taken soon after penetrating the motoneurone. From 5 sec. to

Huxley, 1952c). According to the hypothesis, the rising phase of the spike is caused by the initial inward movement of Na^+ ions along their electrochemical gradient, while the falling phase is caused by the subsequent outward movement of K^+ ions along their electrochemical gradient. If, as in other cells where measurement is possible, the intracellular concentration of Na^+ ions is only about one tenth of the extracellular concentration (cf. Table 1), the equilibrium potential for Na^+ ions will be about +60 mV, i.e., with the interior of the neurone 60 mV positive to the exterior. The steep rising phase of the spike with reversal of the membrane potential is attributable to the intense net inward flux of Na^+ ions, which causes the membrane potential to approach the equilibrium potential for Na^+ ions. The intracellular injection of 25 p. equiv. of Na^+ ions would cause a very large diminution of the concentration difference across the membrane and hence account for the much slower rising phase of the spikes at 25 sec. in Figure 26A. Its lower voltage would be explained both by the lowered equilibrium potential for Na^+ ions resulting from this change in concentration and by the diminution of membrane potential which is normally observed. Similarly, the slower falling phase of the spike in Figure 26A is attributable to the lowered internal concentration of K^+ ions with the consequent diminution in the outward flux of K^+ ions during the phase of high K^+ ion permeability. It is significant that the slow rising phase seen in Figure 26A is a prominent feature only when there is an increased internal Na^+ concentration, while the slow falling phase occurs whenever the internal K^+ concentration is diminished, as in Figure 27F,G.

---

300 sec. the resting potential climbed from −82 mV to −86 mV and was at the latter value for the top record in *B*. For the subsequent four pairs of records in B and C the resting potentials were approx. −74 mV (5 sec. to 15 sec.), −77 mV (75 sec. to 90 sec.), −87 mV (300 sec. to 360 sec.), and −93 mV (600 sec. to 620 sec.). In B and C, a full action potential has been set up in each sweep, although the spike is not shown with the slow sweep and high amplification used to display the after-hyperpolarization. Voltage scale applies to different parts of the figure as indicated (Coombs, Eccles, and Fatt, 1955a).

In Figure 26A the slow recovery back to normal indicates that there has been an extrusion of the excess of Na⁺ ions and a replacement of the lost K⁺ ions. The extrusion of the Na⁺ ions occurs against the electrochemical gradi-

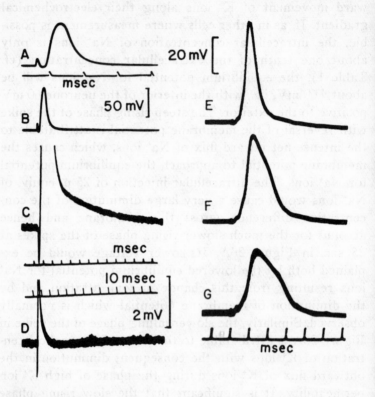

Figure 27

A–D. Intracellular recordings from a motor axon of a single antidromic impulse, each record being formed by superposition of about forty faint traces. Spike responses in A and B are at sweep speeds indicated by millisecond scales below A and C respectively. Potential is given by upper scale. C and D give after-potentials at the much higher amplification shown by lower potential scale. C is at same sweep speed as B, while slower sweep for D is shown by 10 msec. scale. Note that the after-depolarization in C and D persists for about 15 msec., while in D the after-hyperpolarization is very small (about 30 μV) and cannot be detected beyond 80 msec. E. Antidromic spike potentials in a motoneurone on dosage with choline ions. Record E was obtained soon after penetrating the cell and before any injection of ions by current. Resting potential was about −60 mV. Following this, rather less than 10 p. equiv. of choline⁺ (applying 1.5 x 10⁻⁸A for 60 sec.) was injected into

ent and hence must be due to the operation of the sodium pump. The absorption of K$^+$ ions could be due in part to diffusion along the electrochemical gradient, but it will be seen below that in part the potassium pump must be concerned because the normal internal potassium concentration is about double the equilibrium concentration.

The explanation of the ionic mechanism responsible for the spike response of motoneurones would differ in one respect from that proposed by Hodgkin and Huxley (1952c) for spikes in giant axons. With the motoneurone it must be assumed that the high potassium permeability is a sequel of the initial high sodium permeability *per se*, for mere depolarization does not in itself cause a high potassium conductance as it does with giant axons (cf. Chapter I).

It has been shown that the membrane potential of a motoneurone is set at about -70 mV because of the small excess (2×10^{-15} equiv.) of internal anions. Since a motoneuronal spike potential is probably as high as 110 mV if recorded without loss by capacitative distortion (cf. Brock *et al.*, 1952a), the rising phase of the spike would require the net inward movement of at least 3×10^{-15} equiv. of Na$^+$ ions, so giving a small excess of cations, while during the falling phase of the spike the initial excess of anions would be restored by the net outward movement of over 3×10^{-15} equiv. of K$^+$ ions. With giant axons there is such a large overlap in the time courses of these fluxes that the actual net fluxes are two to three times the minimum required for producing the membrane potential change (cf. Hodgkin, 1951). The brevity of the spike suggests that this situation also obtains for motoneurones, hence the net fluxes of Na$^+$ and of K$^+$ ions during the spike would be of the order of 5 to 10×10^{-15} equiv.

---

the cell, and record F was obtained within one minute of the end of the injection. The resting potential remained at -60 mV. After another few minutes the resting potential had fallen to -45 mV and record G was then obtained (Coombs, Eccles, and Fatt, 1955a).

11. The After-Hyperpolarization

a. Voltage and time course

The SD spike potential is always followed by a prolonged period of hyperpolarization, which hitherto has been called the positive after-potential. This term is now a misnomer, however, because the recorded intracellular potential, i.e., the specified potential, actually becomes more negative; hence it will be renamed the "after-hyperpolarization." It is important to discriminate between two motoneuronal hyperpolarizations that are generated by impulses in motor axons. One is the true after-hyperpolarization which is a sequel of the SD spike *per se*. The other is an inhibitory postsynaptic potential that is generated by impulses in motor axons operating through a pathway from motor-axon collaterals to Renshaw cells (cf. Figures 66, 67, 68; Eccles, Fatt, and Koketsu, 1954). With antidromic activation the discrimination is secured easily by employing a stimulus that is just at threshold for the axon of the motoneurone under observation. Thus, as in Figure 28A, two sets of records are obtained according to whether the axon is or is not excited, the difference between them being attributable to the true after-hyperpolarization. This method of discrimination depends on the experimental finding that an impulse in the axon of a motoneurone has a negligible inhibitory effect on that motoneurone (Eccles, Fatt, and Koketsu, 1954).

With a normal neurone the SD spike potential does not immediately reverse to give the after-hyperpolarization, but continues as a declining depolarization for several milliseconds (Figures 18 at −77 mV; 26A). The subsequent after-hyperpolarization increases to reach a maximum of about 5 mV at 10 msec. to 15 msec., and thereafter it gradually declines so that it can no longer be detected after about 100 msec. (Figures 26B,C, lowest records; 28A).

According to Frank and Fuortes (1955b) the after-hyperpolarization does not occur after spikes evoked by orthodromic stimulation. The dorsal root volleys which they employed for orthodromic stimulation, however, would have a large polysynaptic excitatory action, which presumably obscured effectively the after-hyperpolarization (cf. Woodbury and Patton, 1952, Figure 3). Such a complication can be avoided by employing afferent volleys from muscle nerves, which can have a purely monosynaptic excitatory action. Under such conditions the spike potential is followed by an after-hyperpolarization identical with that following an antidromic spike potential, allowance being made as above for any superimposed inhibitory potential. The onset of such a hyperpolarization may be seen in Figures 24 and 51J. The similarity of the after-potentials following antidromically and orthodromically evoked spikes already has been illustrated (Brock *et al.*, 1952a, Figure 3E). It should be noted that IS spikes are not followed by any appreciable after-hyperpolarization even when the membrane is depolarized (Coombs *et al.*, 1955a).

An after-hyperpolarization of about the same voltage but longer duration has been observed in amphibian motoneurones (Araki, Otani, and Furukawa, 1953). It also arises after the spike has terminated in a phase of declining depolarization.

b. *Effect of change in intracellular ionic composition*

Since the capacitance of the surface membrane remains remarkably stable even during a spike potential (Cole and Curtis, 1939; Hodgkin *et al.*, 1952), it is reasonable to suppose that, just as with the spike potential, other potential changes generated in the membrane are caused by the movement of ions across it. In attempting to identify these ions a useful procedure has been to investigate the effects produced by changing the intracellular ionic concentrations.

As shown in Figure 26B,C, the after-hyperpolarization is abolished when a considerable fraction of the intracellular potassium is replaced by sodium. The subsequent recovery follows much the same time course as the recovery of the spike potential.

This effect cannot be attributed to the increased intracellular sodium, because, if the after-hyperpolarization is produced by an increase in sodium movement across the surface membrane, an increased intracellular concentration should cause an increase in the outward movement of sodium, and hence an increase in the after-hyperpolarization. On the other hand, if the after-hyperpolarization is due to an increased movement of K^+ ions across the membrane, its abolition or diminution by depletion of intracellular potassium is to be expected. This suggestion is strengthened further by finding that the after-hyperpolarization is similarly changed when depletion of intracellular potassium is coupled with injection of a cation other than sodium—the tetramethylammonium ion. Since injection of a wide variety of anions into the neurone was without significant effect on the after-hyperpolarization, it may be concluded that it is not associated with an increased permeability to some anions. It therefore stands in sharp contrast to another hyperpolarizing potential—the inhibitory postsynaptic potential (cf. Chapter III).

It thus appears that the after-hyperpolarization is produced entirely by the net outward movement of K^+ ions. Depletion of intracellular potassium reduces this net movement and may even reverse it, as shown by the conversion to an after-depolarization, which has been observed for a short period after a current that produced a very large depletion of the intracellular potassium. The recovery illustrated in Figure 26B,C provides a good means of evaluating the rate of replacement of the lost intracellular potassium. After a moderate depletion, replacement is virtually complete in about 10 minutes.

c. Effect of changes in the membrane potential

If the after-hyperpolarization is thus due solely to the net outward movement of K^+ ions, the effect produced by changing the membrane potential becomes of great significance. If the movement of the K$^+$ ions is due to the operation of a pump, it is unlikely that it would be affected greatly by variation in the membrane potential. At least the sodium pump in giant axons is not affected appreciably by such conditions (Hodgkin and Keynes, 1955). On the other hand, if the movement of the K$^+$ ions is occurring along their electrochemical gradient, it should be changed very effectively, and even reversed, by varying the potential.

Figure 28A shows that the size, but not the time course, of the after-hyperpolarization was greatly changed when the membrane potential was varied by an extrinsic current through one barrel of a double microelectrode, being greatly increased by depolarization and diminished by hyperpolarization. Similar series are illustrated in Figures 4 B–E and 25A. Thus the after-hyperpolarization partly compensates for the changed membrane potential, the compensation being as much as 30 per cent for the series in Figure 28A (cf. Figure 29A). The compensatory effect is illustrated better in Figure 4 B–E, where it is as much as 40 per cent. It was impossible to extend the series of Figure 28A beyond a hyperpolarization to −87 mV, because the antidromic impulse then failed to invade the motoneurone. In Figure 29, however, extrapolation shows that beyond a membrane potential of about −90 mV the after-hyperpolarization should reverse to an after-depolarization. The necessity for extrapolation can be avoided by allowing the antidromic impulses to invade the neurone before applying the hyperpolarizing current pulse. Under such conditions, reversal of the after-hyperpolarization has been observed (Coombs et al., 1955a, Figure 13).

These observations indicate that the after-hyperpolarization is due to the net outward diffusional movement of K$^+$ ions and not to the operation of a potassium pump. Furthermore, they show that the potassium equilibrium potential across the neuronal membrane is about −90 mV (mean of experiments on 7 motoneurones). On the basis of the Nernst equation it therefore becomes possible to

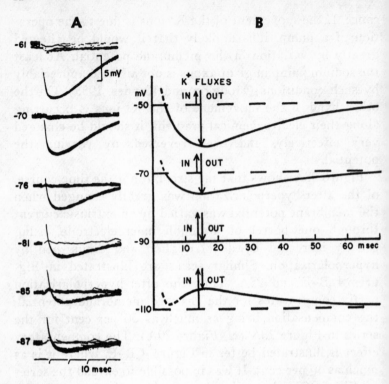

Figure 28

A. After-hyperpolarizations of a motoneurone, occuring at various levels of membrane potential as controlled by extrinsic current. For each record, the stimulus applied to the ventral root was adjusted to the critical strength at which the axon of the particular motoneurone was sometimes excited and other times it was not. The motoneurone was selected because it displayed little inhibitory effect of Renshaw cells (cf. Figure 66) when the stimulus was at the threshold for exciting its axon. The membrane potentials in mV at which the action potentials were evoked are given alongside each record. The resting potential varied from −76 mV to −79 mV. The spike component of the antidromic action potential does not appear in these records, the amplification being too high and the sweep too slow to display it satisfactorily (Coombs, Eccles, and Fatt, 1955a). *B.* Diagrammatic representation of K+ ion fluxes during the after-hyperpolarization that occurs when the membrane potential has been preset at three different levels in addition to the resting potential of −70 mV. The relative diffusional fluxes inward and outward are calculated according to the Nernst equation, and are shown as equal at −90 mV (the equilibrium potential) and with the outward double the inward at −70 mV (cf. Figure 8). The size of the after-hyperpolarization is shown to be directly related to the unbalanced K+ ion flux at −50 mV and −70 mV, while at −90 mV it is zero, and at −110 mV it is converted to an after-

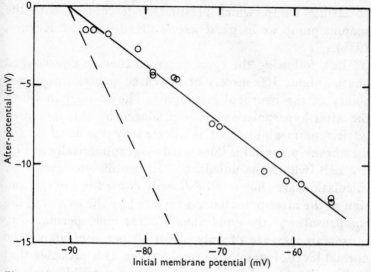

Figure 29

Plot of the peak amplitude of the after-hyperpolarization against membrane potential. Part of the series of records from this motoneurone is illustrated in Figure 28A. A straight line has been fitted to the plotted points. Broken line indicates the relation that would obtain if there was complete compensation by the after-hyperpolarization. Resting potential varied from −76 mV to −79 mV. Negative values of the after-potential indicate increase of internal negativity (Coombs, Eccles, and Fatt, 1955a).

calculate the intracellular concentration of K^+ ions, if the extracellular value is known. Thus,

$$E_K \text{ (in mV)} = 61.5 \log_{10} \frac{(K_o)}{(K_i)},$$

where $E_K = -90$ mV. If the mean value of 5.5 mM for the potassium concentration of an ultrafiltrate of cat plasma is assumed for (K_o) (Coombs *et al.*, 1955b, p. 361), (K_i) is approximately 150 mM. At the normal resting membrane potential of −70 mV, (K_i) would have to be only about 75 mM for diffusional equilibrium, hence (K_i) normally appears to be about twice the equilibrium concentration. This concentration must be built up by the operation of a

---

depolarization because the inward K^+ ion flux is then greater than the outward.

potassium pump, which presumably is coupled with the sodium pump as in giant axons (Hodgkin and Keynes, 1955).

Thus, following the spike potential there is a prolonged phase (about 100 msec.) of increased potassium permeability of the neuronal membrane. The manner in which the after-hyperpolarization is produced by this increased K^+ ion permeability and is affected by the level of the membrane potential is illustrated diagrammatically in Figure 28B, where the unbalanced K^+ ion fluxes, derived by calculation, are shown to be directly related to the size and sign of the after-potential. As revealed by the extent of the compensation, the additional potassium permeability causes an increase of only about 40 per cent above the normal level of membrane conductance. It is probable that such an increase does not require even a doubling of the normal potassium permeability. There is evidence that the prolonged increase in potassium permeability responsible for the after-hyperpolarization can be distinguished from the increased permeability occurring during and just after the decline of the spike potential. When some neurones are subjected to a sufficient depolarization, a phase of partial recovery separates two phases of hyperpolarization. The initial phase continues from the decline of the spike potential, while the second phase is due to the high potassium permeability that gives the after-hyperpolarization. A trace of this separation is seen in Figure 18A at membrane potentials of −60 and −63 mV.

When an antidromic volley is fired into a motor nucleus, a potential attributable to the after-hyperpolarization is observed regularly in records of ventral root potentials (Eccles and Pritchard, 1937; Gasser, 1939; Brooks, Downman and Eccles, 1950a; Lloyd, 1951b). Furthermore, an associated depression of synaptic excitatory action also was observed, its duration of 100 msec. to 120 msec. corresponding closely to that of the after-hyperpolarization. These responses observed in the ventral roots are of significance because they show that the after-hyperpolarization is not secondary to a depolarization of motoneurones that has been brought about by puncture with a microelectrode. For example, if the resting potential were reduced from -90 mV to -70 mV by the puncture, the resting potential would normally equal E_K and there would be no need to assume the operation of a K^+ ion pump. Since the after-hyperpolarization occurs in motoneurones untouched by microelectrodes, this eventuality can be excluded, and it must be assumed that normally E_K is considerably larger than the resting potential.

It is not possible to offer any experimental evidence which leads to an explanation of the brief phase (about 2 msec. to 6 msec.) of depolarization that lies normally between the end of the spike and the onset of the after-hyperpolarization. The equilibrium potential of this depolarizing phase is about -60 mV (cf. Figures 18, 25A). Following the spike of the motor axons in the spinal cord and motor roots there is similarly a phase of after-depolarization (Lloyd, 1951b; J. C. Eccles, 1955), which may be as long as 20 msec. in duration (Figure 27C,D). The longer duration is attributable to the virtual absence of any subsequent after-hyperpolarization.

B. EXCITATORY REACTIONS OF OTHER NERVE CELLS AND SYNAPTIC JUNCTIONS

Other nerve cells have been studied much less intensively than motoneurones. In general, they exhibit responses which are similar qualitatively, though they differ quantitatively, particularly in the duration of the responses, as is illustrated in the following brief accounts.

1. Interneurones in the Spinal Cord

Some intracellular records are available, but usually from neurones with low membrane potentials. Frank and

Fuortes (1955b) illustrate an interneuronal spike potential of about 85 mV and 1 msec. duration that is generated by an EPSP giving 8 mV depolarization. The EPSP set up in an intermediate neurone by a group Ia volley differs from that of motoneurones only in that it may evoke two or more spike discharges from an intermediate neurone (Figure 59 A–C). Single volleys in other types of afferent fibres often evoke prolonged repetitive discharges from interneurones, so it is likely that they set up even more prolonged EPSP's (cf. Figure 70 A–C). The significance of this will be discussed in Chapter VI.

2. Renshaw Cells in the Spinal Cord

The responses of these special interneurones will be described and discussed in Chapter V. With intracellular recording (Figure 64 F–H), the membrane potential and spike potential have been respectively as high as -60 mV and 70 mV, while the spike duration is about 0.5 msec. (Frank and Fuortes, 1956a; Eccles, Fatt, and Koketsu, 1954). The EPSP produced by a single presynaptic volley (in the motor-axon collaterals) takes over 50 msec. to decline from a very early summit (Figure 64I). During this time the Renshaw cell may discharge a series of impulses which are initially at high frequency (up to 1700 a sec.) and thereafter become progressively less frequent (Figure 64). After dosage with anticholinesterases a single presynaptic volley may set up a discharge for as long as 3 sec. (Figure 65D). The initial high-frequency discharge is probably produced in the initial segment of the Renshaw cell which is depolarized very effectively by currents flowing into the soma. Occasionally it is found that with a microelectrode in the soma there appears to be virtually an intermission of one impulse (Figure 64H) during the initial high-frequency phase. Presumably that impulse failed to propagate back into the soma from the axon where it was initiated.

3. Synaptic Relays in the Cuneate Nucleus

There are still virtually no intracellular records for this important synaptic relay. It has been shown, however, that a single presynaptic volley in the dorsal column causes a cuneate neurone to discharge two or three impulses at a frequency as high as 1000 per sec. (Amassian and DeVito, 1956). Since interneurones do not appear to be involved in this discharge, it may be presumed that a prolonged EPSP is responsible for this repetitive discharge, just as with some neurones of the intermediate nucleus; but it is also likely that some delayed excitatory action may be exerted by impulses in recurrent collaterals from the axons of cuneate neurones.

4. Pyramidal Cells in the Cerebral Cortex

By intracellular recording the resting potential has been shown to be about −60 mV (Phillips, 1955; 1956a), while the spike potential may be 80 mV or more (Figure 30A). Synaptic stimulation appears to produce depolarization, which, if adequate, causes the discharge of an impulse (Figure 30B; Li and Jasper, 1953; Jung, 1953b; Albe-Fessard and Buser, 1955; Phillips, 1956a). The spike potential is about 1 msec. in duration and appears to resemble that of the motoneurone both by a notch on the rising phase and by a prolonged after-hyperpolarization (Phillips, 1956a, b). With rapid repetitive responses, some of the spikes may be greatly reduced (Figure 30D), suggesting that IS spikes are produced under such conditions as in Figure 19F,G, and J.

5. Sympathetic Ganglion Cells

When recorded intracellularly (R. M. Eccles, 1955; 1956), a presynaptic volley sets up an excitatory postsynaptic potential of the ganglion cell which is analogous to that of motoneurones, but much slower in time course, having a rising phase of 4 msec. to 9 msec. and a time constant of decay of 6 msec. to 12 msec. This EPSP may be revealed uncomplicated by a spike potential if it is diminished below the threshold level for generating a spike (15 mV to 25 mV), either by decreasing the size of the presynaptic volley (Figure 31 A–D), or by soaking the preparation in a solution of a curarizing agent (Figure 31 F–I). The spike set up antidromically resembles that of motoneurones in

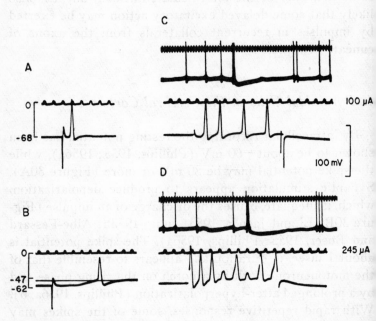

Figure 30

Intracellular records from cells of cat cerebral cortex, *A, C,* and *D* being from large pyramidal cells of the motor cortex (Betz cells). *A* and *B* show spike responses evoked by antidromic and synaptic stimulation respectively in two different cells. Note the gradual depolarization that precedes the spike in *B*. *C* and *D* show responses to rectangular current pulses (surface positive) of 10 msec. duration (100 μA in C and 245 μA in D), which are applied through a stimulating electrode on the cortical surface above the cell. The upper record shows a very slow trace (10-msec. time wave), while the middle portion, which includes the pulse, is displayed in the lower trace at much faster sweep (1-msec. time wave). (Phillips, 1956a,b).

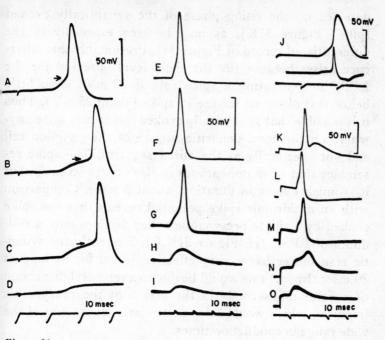

Figure 31

Intracellular records from ganglion cells of the isolated superior cervical ganglion of the rabbit. A is the action potential in response to a maximal single preganglionic volley, and *B, C,* and *D* the responses when the stimulus strength is reduced. Arrows indicate the level of depolarization (14.5 mV) at which the spike arises. *E–I* show a progressive series of potentials evoked by a maximum preganglionic volley, *E* before and *F–I* at intervals of a few minutes (4, 5, 7, and 9 respectively) after addition of a blocking dose of dihydro-β-erythroidine hydrobromide to the bathing solution, the concentration being about 1 in 50,000. The resting membrane potential remained constant at about -66 mV during the whole series. In J the differentiated record below the action potential set up by a preganglionic volley shows that there is no trace of an IS-SD separation. In another ganglion cell, *L* and *M* show the IS-SD separation for antidromic excitation, but not for presynaptic excitation K. With deterioration of another cell there is failure of IS-SD antidromic propagation between *N* and *O* responses (R. M. Eccles, 1955, 1956).

showing a notch on the rising phase at about 20 mV to 30 mV (Figure 31L,M), which likewise may be taken to indicate that a preliminary IS spike precedes the soma-dendritic invasion. On the other hand no notch can be detected on the rising phase of the synaptically evoked spike (Figure 31K), as may be seen especially in the differentiated record of Figure 31J. Presumably this difference arises because the threshold level observed for the EPSP in generating a spike (about 20 mV) is so little below that observed for the IS spike (about 25 mV). Thus it is possible that synaptically evoked spikes may arise anywhere on the soma-dendritic surface of the ganglion cell and not specifically at the initial segment. The spike resembles that of motoneurones in size (up to 95 mV), but it is much longer in duration, about 5 msec. Comparison with an antidromic spike potential reveals that the spike evoked by a single presynaptic volley declines onto a residuum of EPSP (cf. Figure 31K,L). Evidently the synaptic transmitter has a very effective action for as long as 20 msec. In part this would be due to a temporal dispersion of several milliseconds in the action of the presynaptic impulses, which would arise particularly on account of the wide range in conduction times.

6. Stretch Receptor Cells of Crustacean Muscle

These large receptor cells were first described by Alexandrowicz (1951, 1952) and then were extensively investigated physiologically by Wiersma, Furshpan, and Florey (1953). More recently Eyzaguirre and Kuffler (1955a,b) have studied their responses by intracellular recording, but unfortunately no excitatory synaptic action has yet been detected. A cell can be excited to discharge impulses (Figures 32C,D, 57), however, if its dendrites are depolarized sufficiently by stretching the muscle fibres in which they are embedded (Figure 49A). The normal resting membrane potential of the cell is −70 mV to −80 mV, and the threshold depolarization is about 20 mV and 10 mV for the fast adapting and slow adapting cells respectively, subthreshold depolarizations being shown in Figure 32A,B. The threshold depolarization, however, may be considerably

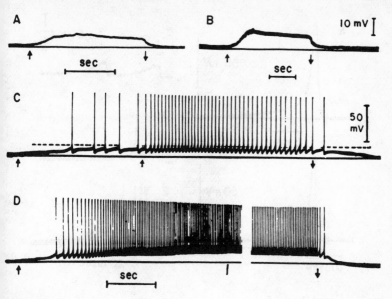

Figure 32

Membrane potential changes of crustacean stretch receptor cells recorded intracellularly (cf. Figure 49A) and produced by the application of stretches which were applied between the upward and downward pointing arrows. In *A* and *B,* the stretches of the receptor organs were too small to evoke the discharge of impulses from slow and fast adapting cells respectively. In *C* and *D,* larger stretches evoked repetitive discharges from a slowly adapting cell. The frequency in *C* increased up to 12 to 14 per sec. when a further stretch was applied at the second upward arrow, but the "firing level" of depolarization remained almost constant at the level indicated by the broken line. In *D,* the frequency increased up to 30 per sec. during a gradual increment in stretch and it continued at about 30 per sec. during maintained stretch, several seconds of the record being omitted at the gap (Eyzaguirre and Kuffler, 1955a).

higher at the actual site of origin of the impulses, which may be in the dendrites some distance from the soma.

If an impulse propagates antidromically down the afferent axon, it may invade the receptor cell and evoke a spike response of 70 mV to 90 mV and about 2 msec. in duration. If the membrane potential is at the fully relaxed value, the spike declines onto a slowly decaying depolarization (Figure 33A). If, on the other hand, the membrane is depolarized, the spike is followed immediately by a large

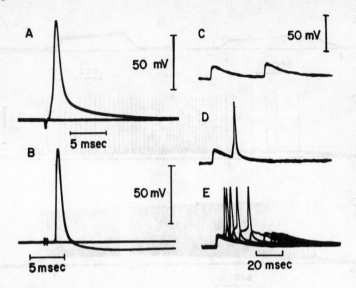

Figure 33

Membrane potential changes recorded intracellularly and generated by firing impulses antidromically along the axons of slowly adapting stretch receptor cells of crustacea. Single antidromic impulses produced response A in the cell of a relaxed stretch receptor (resting potential, −70 mV) and response B in the cell when its resting potential was reduced to −60 mV by application of a light stretch to the receptor organ. C – E show responses of a relaxed cell (membrane potential, −70 mV) to two antidromic impulses at various intervals, there being in E superimposed records over a wide range of intervals (Eyzaguirre and Kuffler, 1955b).

after-hyperpolarization (Figure 33B), just as occurs with depolarized motoneurones (cf. Figures 4D,E, and upper records of 18A, 25A). Alternatively the antidromic impulse may be blocked at the axon-soma junction, or there might be partial invasion giving local responses. Even in the absence of such local responses, however, a blocked impulse usually causes a fairly prolonged depolarization of the soma, the time constant of the approximately exponential decay being as much as 20 msec. (Figure 33C). During this prolonged depolarization there is facilitation that may enable a second antidromic impulse to invade the cell (Figure 33D,E). With other cells a blocked impulse may cause a relatively brief depolarization of the soma, much as with the IS spike of motoneurones. Facilitation then is not observed. It is noteworthy that, in contrast with motoneurones, there is, with fast adapting cells, much the same threshold of depolarization (about 20 mV) for antidromic invasion of the soma and for the generation of impulses by stretch depolarization. Apparently, as with sympathetic ganglion cells, the threshold depolarization for the soma is much the same as that for the axon. This difference from motoneurones might arise because the stretch receptor cell is not covered by synaptic knobs as is the soma of a motoneurone.

7. Giant Synapses of Stellate Ganglion of Loligo

As shown in Figure 34A, a second order giant fibre makes a very extensive synaptic contact with the surface of a third order giant fibre in the stellate ganglion, as described by Young (1939). With extracellular recording, Bullock (1948) showed that transmission through this synapse had the characteristic properties of synaptic delay of about 0.5 msec. (24°C); and, if transmission was blocked by fatigue, a presynaptic impulse still produced a postsynaptic potential. This synapse is unique because the very large size of the presynaptic and postsynaptic structures (Figure 34A) allows the simultaneous recording both of the presynaptic spike and of the postsynaptic response by means of intracellular electrodes (Bullock and Hagiwara, 1956). It is found that the presynaptic spike is virtually over before the onset of the postsynaptic response, there being an interval of 0.5 msec. between the respective onsets at 22°C (2.0 msec. at 10°C). As shown in Figure 34B, a trace of the presynaptic spike may be recorded postganglionically but often (Figure 34C) it can not be detected. Both these figures show that the initial spike transmission was reduced to a postsynaptic potential during repetitive stimulation. These records are particularly convincing in establishing that transmission across

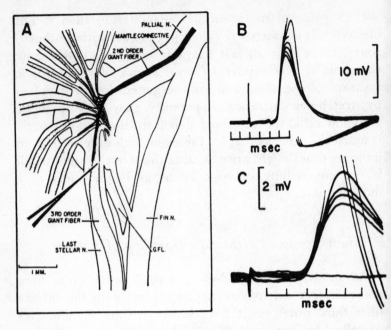

Figure 34

A. Diagram of stellate ganglion in *Loligo* to show synapses between a second order giant fibre and the third order giant fibres. The approximate position of the intracellular microelectrode is indicated in the third order giant fibre of the last stellar nerve just below the synaptic region (modified from Young, 1939, and Bullock, 1948). *B, C.* Intracellular recording as shown in Figure 34A of response evoked by an impulse in the second order giant fibre. Note in B the very small diphasic spike (about 2 msec. after the stimulus artefact) produced by the field recording of this impulse. During repetitive stimulation in B and C there is a progressive delay and eventually blockage of transmission of impulses across the synapse, so that the underlying excitatory postsynaptic potential is revealed, in the last records of the superimposed traces (Bullock and Hagiwara, 1956).

the giant synapse has a synaptic delay and is not due to the flow of electric current. Presumably, as with other synapses, a chemical transmitter mechanism is involved. Figure 34B,C further shows that the EPSP has a rising phase of 1 msec. to 2 msec. and its decay is approximately exponential with a time constant of about 1.2 msec. in Figure 34B. Since the time constant of the postsynaptic fibre is about 1.0 msec. (Hodgkin, 1951), it is evident that the synaptic transmitter must be removed very rapidly from the site of its action.

8. Motor Neurones of the Electric Lobe of Torpedo

The responses of these neurones have been recorded intracellularly. By electrical stimulation of the spinal cord it has been possible to excite them synaptically (Albe-Fessard and Buser, 1954). Subliminal excitation produces a brief wave of depolarization, up to 15 mV in amplitude and about 6 msec. duration, which is essentially an excitatory postsynaptic potential. With supraliminal excitation, this wave is seen as a prepotential from which arises a spike potential of 60 mV to 65 mV and a duration of about 1 msec. However, there is often a transitional phase with partial spike responses, which may be comparable with the responses seen in deteriorated motoneurones (cf. Figure 19 L–O).

9. Ganglion Cells of Aplysia

Tauc (1955a,b) has recorded the potentials which are produced in these large ganglion cells by synaptic excitation. With subthreshold excitation the EPSP resembles other EPSP's except for its extraordinarily long time course, the time to summit being 100 msec. or more, while the time constant of decay is at least 500 msec. Tauc suggests that, since the decay of the EPSP is many times slower than after a depolarization produced by extrinsic current, the chemical transmitter is acting throughout the whole duration of the EPSP. A very effective transmitter action of many seconds' duration is also indicated by the finding that propagation of an impulse over the surface of the cell inactivates a relatively small fraction of the EPSP, which is in contrast with the situation with motoneurones (cf. Figure 12). The threshold level of the EPSP varies greatly in different cells, the range being from 8 mV to 40 mV. The spike potential initiated by the EPSP often rises in two phases, much as occurs with motoneurones. Possibly there is some low threshold area of the ganglion cell corresponding to the initial axonal segment of motoneurones. The spike potential of up to 100 mV is no longer than 10 msec. in duration and it is followed by a prolonged and large after-hyperpolarization.

C. SUMMARY

Intracellular recording from a wide variety of nerve cells has revealed remarkable parallels in the essential features of synaptic transmission. There is general agreement that the synaptic excitation of all nerve cells evokes a depolarization of the postsynaptic membrane (the EPSP) which generates an impulse if it is sufficiently intense. In this action, it can sum with the depolarizations produced by preceding or concurrent impulses or by an extrinsic current. There is no evidence that synaptic excitation is effective by any means other than through the mediation of an excitatory postsynaptic potential. In general, nerve cells have spike potentials that are considerably longer in duration than those of their axons. So far as investigated, these potentials appear to be generated by an ionic mechanism resembling that of axons. There is general agreement also that the electric currents produced by the presynaptic impulses have no detectable effect on the postsynaptic membrane. Synaptically induced depolarization does not begin until the presynaptic spike potential is virtually over, as is demonstrated particularly well by the simultaneous intracellular recording from the presynaptic and postsynaptic components of the giant synapses of *Loligo* (Bullock and Hagiwara, 1956).

Evidently synaptic excitatory action is mediated by chemical transmitters which act on the subsynaptic membrane and cause an inward current to flow across it. The problems relating to transmitter substances themselves will be dealt with in Chapters V and VI. The available evidence suggests that excitatory transmitter substances make the synaptic membrane permeable to a wide variety of ions, both anions and cations, and it thus acts as a virtual short-circuit for current flowing from the remainder of the postsynaptic membrane, just as occurs at the neuromuscular junction. This depolarizing subsynaptic current usually has a very brief duration, presumably because the transmitter is rapidly removed from the subsynaptic membrane. The time courses of the EPSP's indicate that the transmitters have effective durations varying from 1 msec. to 10 msec. for most of the nerve cells so far investigated. Notable exceptions are provided by the giant ganglion cells of *Aplysia*, where the duration is several seconds, and by the Renshaw cells in the spinal cord, where it is normally about 50 msec., though it may be as long as 3 sec. when the cholinesterase is inactivated. Evidently there are here special devices for limiting the rate of diffusion of the transmitter substances from the synaptic regions (cf. Chapter VI). Probably other synapses resemble those on motoneurones, where the effective transmitter action is very brief, and the relatively slow decay of the unitary EPSP is attributable largely to the electric time constant of the postsynaptic membrane.

There are considerable variations between the different types of nerve cells in respect to the threshold level of depolarization for generating a spike potential, and the thresholds for the various regions of the cells. With motoneurones the threshold depolarizations are about 10 mV for the initial segment of the axon and 30 mV for the soma-dendritic membrane. There are indications of this differentiation also for other nerve cells, but there is very little threshold differentiation for the sympathetic ganglion cells. Much more investigation is required before generalizations can be made. Usually the threshold level of depolarization has been within the range, 10 mV to 20 mV.

There is also a wide variation in the after-potentials following a spike potential. For example, at the resting membrane potential the crustacean stretch receptor cell shows no after-hyperpolarization, and after-hyperpolarization is inconspicuous with interneurones of the spinal cord. On the other hand, motoneurones and cortical pyramidal cells exhibit after-hyperpolarizations of considerable size and up to 100 msec. in duration. Probably the after-hyperpolarizations exhibited by all types of nerve cells are caused by an increased permeability to K^+ ions, as has been demonstrated for motoneurones. The crustacean stretch receptor cell exhibits no after-hyperpolarization when it is in the relaxed state because the ionic mechanism is in equilibrium. The displacement from this equilibrium by depolarization causes a large after-hyperpolarization (Figure 33B). Similarly with other types of nerve cell there may be no after-hyperpolarization because normally the ionic mechanism is in equilibrium. Alternatively, in some varieties of nerve cells, the spike potential may not induce a prolonged phase of selective ionic permeability. For example, no appreciable after-hyperpolarization has been observed with interneurones of the spinal cord even when they were heavily depolarized, and the IS spike is not followed by an after-hyperpolarization even when the motoneurone is heavily depolarized (Coombs *et al.*, 1955a). This remarkable difference between the after-potentials given by the membranes responsible for the IS and SD spikes may derive from the same intrinsic difference in membrane properties that was postulated in explanation of the three-fold ratio of thresholds.

CHAPTER III

THE INHIBITORY REACTIONS
OF NERVE CELLS

Until recently the only criterion of inhibitory synaptic activity was the depression of a testing reflex discharge. When a conditioning volley or train of impulses in one afferent nerve was found to depress a testing reflex response evoked by impulses in another afferent nerve, it was said to exert an inhibitory action. Some of these so-called inhibitory actions can be explained by the depression which is exhibited by a neurone after it has discharged an impulse (cf. Figures 12, 19A–J), or even after a post-synaptic response that is subliminal for generating an impulse. Such an eventuality, however, can be readily detected and avoided if a monosynaptic reflex is employed for testing (cf. Lloyd, 1941b; 1946; Renshaw, 1942). Strictly, the concept of inhibition is restricted to depressions of neuronal reflex excitability which occur independently of conditioning excitatory synaptic activity on that neurone, and also independently of any depression of the excitatory synaptic bombardment that is employed in testing for the suspected inhibition.

Various explanations have been given for this fundamental kind of nervous activity, but the experimental data were necessarily too indirect to permit rigorous testing and discrimination (cf. Brooks and Eccles, 1948). This unsatisfactory position no longer exists. It has been shown that inhibitory actions on motoneurones are explained satisfactorily by the transient increases which are produced in their membrane potentials and which have been designated inhibitory postsynaptic potentials, IPSP (Brock *et al.*, 1952a; Coombs *et al.*, 1955b,d).

Similarly it has been shown that the synaptic inhibitory action on crustacean stretch receptor cells is attributable to a repolarizing action which is exerted on cells that have been depolarized by stretch (Kuffler and Eyzaguirre, 1955). Related inhibitory mechanisms have also been described for other junctional regions, the crustacean neuromuscular junction (Fatt and Katz, 1953) and the vagal action on the heart (Castillo and Katz, 1955c; Hutter and Trautwein, 1955), while it is also possible that a comparable inhibitory action is exerted on some sympathetic ganglion cells (Laporte and Lorente de Nó, 1950; Lorente de Nó and Laporte, 1950; R. M. Eccles, 1956).

Since the inhibitory responses of mammalian motoneurones have been investigated more completely, they will be described fully before giving an account of the other inhibitory phenomena.

A. MOTONEURONES

Five different types of inhibitory action have been investigated and have been found to exhibit virtually identical behaviour under all tests; hence the present account will be restricted to the two types that are most suitable for investigation because they may be obtained uncomplicated by synaptic excitatory action: the so-called direct inhibitory action which is exerted on motoneurones of antagonistic muscles by the large group I afferent fibres from the annulospiral endings, one interneurone being interpolated in the pathway (Eccles, Fatt, and Landgren, 1956); and the so-called antidromic inhibitory action exerted by impulses in motor-axon collaterals, again by way of an interneurone (Eccles, Fatt, and Koketsu, 1954).

Little complication is produced by the interneuronal linkage in the direct inhibitory pathway because a single primary afferent volley evokes only a single discharge from most of the interneurones. It should be stated further that, by using the threshold discrimination between group Ia and group Ib of quadriceps afferent fibres (cf. Bradley and Eccles, 1953), it has been possible to evoke, in biceps-semitendinosus motoneurones, direct inhibitory responses which are virtually uncomplicated by effects produced by quadriceps group Ib impulses (cf. Laporte and Lloyd, 1952).

By way of contrast, a single volley in the motor-axon collaterals evokes a prolonged repetitive discharge from the interneurone (Figure 64), with the consequence that the IPSP is correspondingly prolonged, though it has the advantage of being uncontaminated by any EPSP response.

The time course of the IPSP produced by the direct inhibitory action of a single volley thus approximates to that produced by a single impulse at a single synapse, while the more prolonged IPSP's produced by other types of inhibitory action may be assumed to be produced both by a temporal dispersion of many milliseconds in the activation of the inhibitory synapses and by the repetitive activation of these synapses. In addition to antidromic inhibition these more prolonged IPSP's arise with the inhibitions produced by group Ib muscle afferents (Granit, 1950; Granit and Ström, 1951; Laporte and Lloyd, 1952), by group II and III muscle afferents, and by cutaneous afferents (cf. Renshaw, 1942; Hagbarth, 1952).

1. Intracellular Recording of the Inhibitory Postsynaptic Potential, IPSP

As shown in Figure 35 a single group Ia volley in quadriceps afferent fibres evokes a hyperpolarizing response (the IPSP) in a motoneurone of the antagonist muscle (biceps-semitendinosus), the membrane potential of −66 mV being increased to over −68 mV. The inhibitory pathway by way of an intermediate neurone is shown in Figures 62 and 63. In Figure 35 the IPSP increased in

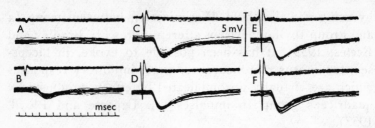

Figure 35

Lower records give intracellular responses of a biceps-semitendinosus motoneurone to a quadriceps volley of progressively increasing size, as is shown by the upper records which are recorded from the L6 dorsal root by a surface electrode (downward deflections signalling negativity). Note three gradations in the size of the IPSP; from *A* to *B,* from *B* to *C* and from *D* to *E.* All records are formed by the superposition of about forty faint traces. Voltage scale gives 5 mV for intracellular records, downward deflexions indicating membrane hyperpolarization. (Coombs, Eccles, and Fatt, 1955d).

three stages with increase in the size of the afferent volley, but the time course remained virtually unchanged. Just as with the EPSP it may be concluded that each inhibitory synapse generates a potential response of this same time course, and that the recorded potentials of Figure 35 are produced by summation of these elemental inhibitory potentials. Within a single motoneurone there is thus spatial summation of inhibitory as well as of excitatory activity (cf. Sherrington, 1925).

With direct inhibitory action the IPSP has been observed to begin as soon as 1.25 msec. after the primary afferent volley has entered the spinal cord, but a minimum central latency of 1.5 msec. is observed when, as in Figure 58B (cf. interval between arrow and IPSP), the inhibitory pathway has a longitudinal component as large as 15 mm (Eccles, Fatt, and Landgren, 1956). The IPSP reaches its summit about 1.5 msec. to 2 msec. after its onset, and thereafter an approximately exponential decay eventuates, the mean time constant for a large number of experiments being about 3.0 msec. Thus the IPSP is approximately a mirror image of the EPSP, differing in its longer latency and in the shorter time constant of decay. It also differs in that it declines to the original base-line with no trace of the overshoot observed with the EPSP (cf. Figure 10D,E).

2. The Current That Flows during the IPSP

In order to produce the observed hyperpolarization, current must be flowing inward across the motoneuronal membrane in general, and there must be a corresponding outward current in the region of the activated inhibitory synapses. Our present problem is to determine the time course of the current and the changes produced in the current by variations in the membrane potential. As was done with the EPSP (Figures 20, 21), and with the same reservations, it should be possible to determine in this way the equilibrium potential for the current that generates the IPSP.

The time course of the current that produces the IPSP may be determined from the IPSP if the time constant of the membrane is known. The broken line of Figure 36A plots the time course so determined, and shows that the high intensity phase has virtually the same time course as the excitatory subsynaptic current (Figure 11B). The maximum intensity is attained in about 0.5 msec., after which there is a rapid decline. In contrast to the EPSP, however, there is little or no residual current after 2 msec. The slight and transient reversal of current in Figure 36A at this time is presumably attributable to the current that causes the electrotonic spread of the IPSP from the soma to the axon and the more remote regions of the dendrites. The negligible size of the residual current may be correlated with the finding that the mean time constant of decay of the IPSP (3.0 msec.) is only slightly longer than the mean value for the electric time constant of the motoneuronal membrane (2.5 msec.).

Two other types of investigation have also provided evi-

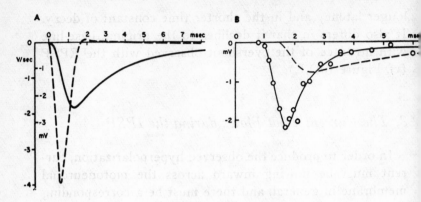

Figure 36

A. Continuous line plots the mean time course of the IPSP set up in a biceps-semitendinosus motoneurone by a single quadriceps Ia volley. The measured time constant for the membrane was 2.8 msec. The broken line gives the time course of the inhibitory subsynaptic current that would produce the IPSP, the calculation being similar to that used in deriving Figure 11A. *B.* Open circles plot the diminution produced in the summit of the antidromic spike potential of a motoneurone when it is set up at various times relative to an IPSP (shown by the broken line). Abscissae give the times of onset of the antidromic spikes relative to the arrival of the directly inhibiting quadriceps volley at the spinal cord. Spike summits were about 0.5 msec. later (Coombs, Eccles, and Fatt, 1955d).

dence that the ionic conductance of the subsynaptic membrane is changed with approximately the time course of Figure 36A.

(i) When a testing antidromic volley was set up at various times before and during an IPSP, it was found that it was considerably diminished in size if the rising phase of the spike coincided with the rising phase of the IPSP. As shown in Figure 36B the maximum depression occurred when the spike summit was late on the rising phase of the IPSP, and a considerable depression was observed for a range of volley intervals extending over little more than 2 msec., after which there still was a small depression. This depression of the antidromic spike potential was produced even when dosage by Cl⁻ ions had converted the IPSP to a depolarizing response. It may be concluded that the depression is caused by the high ionic conductance which obtains especially during the first two milliseconds of the IPSP and which will be shown later to be causally related to the subsynaptic current.

(ii) It will also be shown later that interaction with an EPSP provides evidence for this initial phase of high ionic conductance, and possibly also for a small residual effect (Figures 54B, 55I).

The IPSP is greatly modified by relatively small changes in membrane potential, being increased by depolarization, and diminished or even reversed by hyperpolarization (Figures 37A–G, 38A–G). Plotting of the series of observations partly illustrated in these figures shows that at about −80 mV both types of IPSP changed from a hyperpolarizing to a depolarizing response (Figure 39; cf. also Figures 44, 45). In fact the IPSP can be regarded as being produced by a current across the postsynaptic membrane which tends to bring its voltage to −80 mV. The further the membrane potential is removed from this equilibrium potential of −80 mV, the larger is the IPSP, and hence presumably the larger is its generating current.

In determining the equilibrium potential for the postsynaptic inhibitory mechanism (the E_{IPSP}), it is important to employ a microelectrode filled with a salt solution having large anions such as sulphate, otherwise abnormally low values would be obtained for the E_{IPSP}, as will be described later. Under such conditions, the E_{IPSP} had a mean value of −78 mV in the eight investigations on direct inhibition and of −80 mV in the seven investigations on antidromic inhibition. It is significant that these values are much lower than the mean value of almost −90 mV for the equilibrium potential of the after-hyperpolarization. This difference indicates that different ionic mechanisms are concerned in producing these two types of hyperpolarization, i.e., that the IPSP cannot be generated simply by the movement of K^+ ions as with the after-hyperpolarization. It will be observed further that normally the inhibitory currents are driven by a voltage of only about 10 mV, which is the difference between the E_{IPSP} at −80 mV and the membrane potential of −70 mV. The effects of variations in the membrane potential on the IPSP are in accord with the postulate that the currents generating the IPSP are produced by ions that are moving down their electrochemical gradients and are not being transported independently of these gradients by pumps.

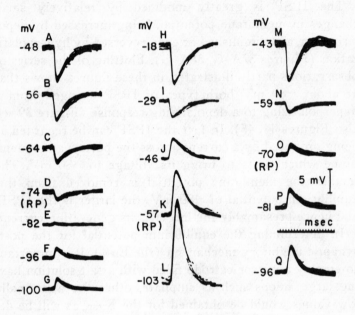

Figure 37

Potentials recorded intracellularly from a biceps-semitendinosus motoneurone by means of a double-barrelled microelectrode filled with Na_2SO_4 (1.2 equiv. per litre). The records, formed by the superposition of about forty faint traces, show the potentials set up by the direct inhibitory action of a group Ia quadriceps afferent volley. By means of a steady background current through one barrel of the double microelectrode, the membrane potential has been preset at the voltage indicated on each record. *A–G* show the IPSP response at the indicated membrane potentials before the passage of a depolarizing current of 5 x 10^{-8}A for 90 sec., and *H–L* immediately (5 sec. to 40 sec.) after. *M–Q* show partial recovery at 180 sec. to 230 sec. In the absence of the background polarizing current, the resting membrane potentials for the three groups of records were −74 mV, −57 mV, and −70 mV, respectively. Potential and time scales apply to all records (Coombs, Eccles, and Fatt, 1955b).

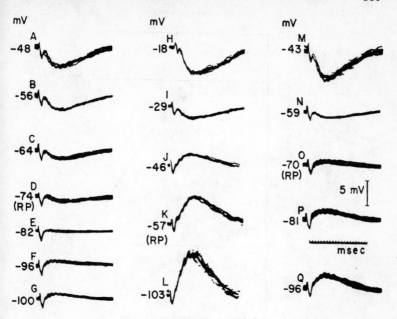

Figure 38

Potentials recorded from the same motoneurone as in Figure 37 and with the same microelectrode, but in this case the response resulted from the inhibitory action evoked by an antidromic volley set up in L7 and S1 ventral roots by a stimulus just below threshold for the axon of the motoneurone. Otherwise, the conditions are the same as for Figure 37. *A–G* show the response before the passage of the depolarizing current of 5 x 10^{-8}A for 90 sec., *H–L* immediately (5 sec to 40 sec.) after, and *M–Q* the partial recovery at 180 sec. to 230 sec. Potential and time scales apply to all records (Coombs, Eccles, and Fatt, 1955b).

3. Effect of Intracellular Injections of Various Ions on the IPSP

We now have to identify the ionic mechanism that at the normal membrane potential causes the inhibitory current to flow across the inhibitory subsynaptic membrane in an outward direction. This outward current could be due to the outward movement of a cation such as potassium, or to the inward movement of an anion like chloride, or to the combined movements of both cations and anions

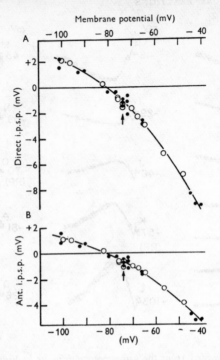

Figure 39

Maximum voltages of the IPSP's of the series partly shown in Figures 37A–G and 38A–G are plotted as ordinates against the respective membrane potentials as abscissae, *A* being for the direct IPSP's and *B* for the antidromic IPSP's. According to the convention adopted throughout this monograph, hyperpolarizing and depolarizing IPSP's are plotted, respectively, as negative and positive voltages. Filled circles were obtained before, and open circles some 9 min. after, the passage of a depolarizing current of 5 x 10^{-8}A for 90 sec. There was no significant change in the resting potential, the mean value being indicated by the arrows (Coombs, Eccles, and Fatt, 1955b).

in these respective directions. All these conditions would increase the small internal excess of anions and so give hyperpolarization.

As already described, it is possible to effect an approximately quantitative injection of a particular ion by passing an electric current through a microelectrode filled with the appropriate salt solution. It is found that the injections of some anion species are particularly effective in modifying the IPSP, but, when microelectrodes filled with such solu-

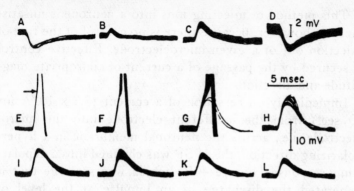

Figure 40

Intracellular recording through a double-barrelled microelectrode filled with 3 M-KCl of IPSP's generated in a biceps-semitendinosus motoneurone by a quadriceps group Ia afferent volley. *A, B,* and *C* show the effect of diffusion of Cl^- ·ions out of the microelectrode in changing the IPSP recorded at the resting membrane potential (-59 mV), while *D* shows restoration of the hyperpolarizing IPSP when the membrane is depolarized by extrinsic current to a lower potential (-27 mV). The voltage scale of D applies to the records *A–D.* Following the passage of a hyperpolarizing current of 3.2×10^{-8}A for 60 sec., the records *E–L* were obtained, all at the resting potential without the application of extrinsic current. By the time of record *L,* recovery was nearly complete, as shown by comparison with record *C.* Spikes in *E, F,* and *G* are truncated. Wide variations in spike latency are shown in *F* and *G.* All records are formed by the super-position of about forty traces (Coombs, Eccles, and Fatt, 1955b).

tions are inserted into a motoneurone, the IPSP changes spontaneously before the effect of a current can be tested. For example, immediately after the insertion of a micro-electrode filled with 3 M KCl, a typical hyperpolarizing IPSP (Figure 40A) changed to the depolarizing responses of Figure 40B,C, and there was little further change thereafter. This change occurred in the absence of any significant alteration in the membrane potential, but, when this potential was diminished to -41 mV, the IPSP was again of the hyperpolarizing type (Figure 40D). The E_{IPSP} had fallen spontaneously to about -50 mV. It will be seen later that this effect is explained sufficiently by postulating that the chloride concentration of the neurone has been increased by diffusion out of the microelectrode.

This method of injecting ions into a neurone is unsatisfactory, however, because there is no control of the rate of injection out of a given microelectrode. Effective control is secured by the passage of a current of appropriate magnitude and direction.

Immediately on cessation of a current (3.2×10^{-8}A for 60 sec.) from the indifferent electrode into the microelectrode, i.e., across the neuronal membrane in a hyperpolarizing direction, the IPSP was changed into a depolarizing response (Figure 40E) which was so large that it generated the discharge of an impulse at the level of depolarization indicated by the arrow (cf. also Figure 40F,G). Recovery toward the initial response (Figure 40C) is shown in the series (Figure 40E–K) at successive intervals of about 10 sec.

Injection of chloride ions into a motoneurone invariably produced this kind of change in the IPSP, converting it into a depolarizing response. This effect is readily ex-

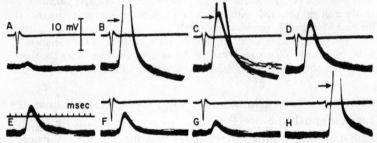

Figure 41

Intracellularly recorded potentials from a biceps-semitendinosus motoneurone with a single microelectrode filled with 3 M-KNO₃. In *A–G*, a quadriceps group Ia afferent volley set up an IPSP, and in H, a biceps-semitendinosus volley set up an EPSP. In *A–D* and *F–H* the surface recorded potentials from the L6 dorsal root are shown above the intracellular record, negativity being downward. A shows the IPSP before, and B immediately after, the passage of a hyperpolarizing current of 3×10^{-8}A for 60 sec. The large depolarizing IPSP sets up a spike in *B* and *C*, the threshold shown by the arrow being about the same as the threshold for the EPSP (arrow in H). All spikes are truncated. Records *C–G* show progressive recovery of the IPSP toward the initial small depolarizing response (A). Potential and time scales apply to all records. (Coombs, Eccles, and Fatt, 1955b).

plained if the movement of Cl⁻ ions across the subsynaptic membrane contributes to the IPSP. For example, the normal hyperpolarizing IPSP could be due to a net inward movement of Cl⁻ ions, which would be converted to a net outward movement and hence a depolarizing IPSP, if the internal concentration of Cl⁻ ions were sufficiently increased. The recovery process was so rapid (half-time about 20 sec.) that with our present technique it was not possible to plot the IPSP/membrane potential curve soon enough after an ionic injection in order to determine the maximum diminution so produced in the E_{IPSP}. However, at 10 sec. to 20 sec. after the current, a diminution of as much as 20 mV to 30 mV has been observed, e.g., from −80 mV down to −55 mV. Similar changes in the IPSP are also produced by injection of some other anion species. For example, the effect of injection of NO_3^- ions and the recovery therefrom is shown in Figure 41. The initial diffusional process had converted the hyperpolarizing IPSP into the small initial depolarizing and the later hyperpolarizing phase shown in Figure 41A, and after the applied hyperpolarizing current the sequence of changes (Figure 41B–G) resembled those of Figure 40. Br⁻ and SCN⁻ ions are similarly effective. The time courses of recovery after NO_3^- and Br⁻ injections are shown in Figure 42 to be approximately exponential with time constants between 25 sec. and 50 sec.

Other anion species such as $SO_4^=$, $HPO_4^=$, $H_2PO_4^-$, HCO_3^-, and CH_3COO^- are ineffective, however, as is illustrated for phosphate (Figure 43A–B) and sulphate (Figure 43E–F) injections. It appears that such species of anions are incapable of contributing to the production of the IPSP. The significance of this difference will be discussed after the effect of cations on the IPSP has been considered. For the present these negative results are of importance in showing that the passage of current in itself does not have as a sequel the changes in the IPSP illustrated in Figures 40, 41, and 42, which must, therefore, be due to the ionic injection produced thereby.

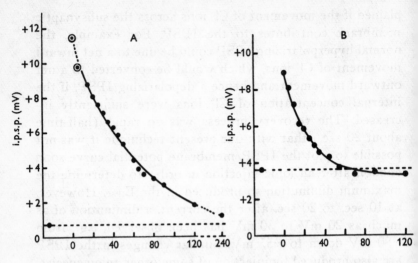

Figure 42

A. Plot of heights of IPSP's, showing time course of recovery after a hyperpolarizing current (3×10^{-8}A for 60 sec.) for the series partly shown in Figure 41. The two points designated ⊙ are the first two responses (cf. Figure 41B) where the spike obscured the summit, the points being calculated from the slopes of the rising phases. The initial point on the horizontal broken line gives the initial response (Figure 41A). *B.* Plot of IPSP's as in *A,* but during recovery after a hyperpolarizing current (4×10^{-8}A for 60 sec.) had been applied through an electrode filled with 4 M-KBr (Coombs, Eccles, and Fatt, 1955b).

An interesting feature of Figures 40 and 41 is that, if the IPSP attains a critical level of depolarization, it generates a spike potential, which also has been observed with the IPSP of crustacean receptor cells (Kuffler and Eyzaguirre, 1955). As shown by comparing Figure 41 B and C with H, the threshold level of depolarization indicated by the horizontal arrows has the same value for the depolarizing IPSP as for the EPSP. This similarity of thresholds is readily explicable because the respective subsynaptic areas are merely providing depolarizing currents for the remainder of the surface membrane of the neurone, including the initial segment, whose response would be determined by the consequent change in potential regardless of any difference which there may be in the ionic

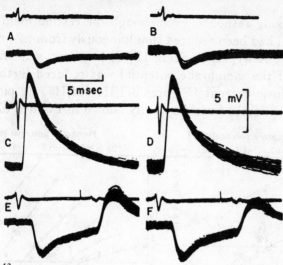

Figure 43

A–D show intracellular potentials recorded with a microelectrode filled with 2 M-(K_2HPO_4 + KH_2PO_4), *A* and *B* being directly evoked IPSP's and *C* and *D* monosynaptic EPSP's. A comparison of *B* with *A* and *D* with *C* indicates that there was no significant change subsequent to the passage of a hyperpolarizing current of 4 x 10^{-8}A for 60 sec. Resting potential constant at −59 mV. For records *E* and *F*, the microelectrode was filled with 0.6 M-K_2SO_4. In each record an IPSP is followed by an EPSP. *E* shows the responses before the passage of a hyperpolarizing current of 4 x 10^{-8}A for 90 sec., and *F* after. There is no significant effect on the IPSP and only a slight depression of the EPSP. The membrane potential was constant at −40 mV. Time and potential scales apply to all the intracellular records (Coombs, Eccles, and Fatt).

mechanisms generating the currents. Since the intracellular microelectrode measures the mean potential change which such currents produce in the neuronal membrane, the same threshold levels of depolarization are to be expected.

The same experimental tests that were employed with the after-hyperpolarization have been used in order to discover if the movements of cations contribute significantly to the IPSP. As shown in Figures 37K and 38K after passing a current of 5 x 10^{-8}A for 90 sec. from a microelectrode filled with Na_2SO_4 solution (1.2 equiv. per litre) to the indifferent electrode, the IPSP was converted to a larger depolarizing response, even though the resting membrane potential had been reduced simultaneously from -74 mV to -57 mV. A hyperpolarizing IPSP, however, was still observed if the membrane potential was reduced further by an extrinsic current (Figures 37I,H; 38I,H). By plotting the series of observations partly shown in Figures 37H–L

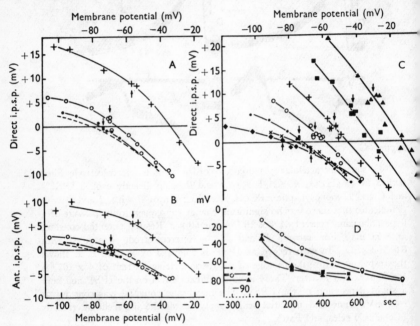

Figure 44

A. Points designated + and ○ plot the series partly shown in Figure 37H–L and M–Q, respectively, on the same co-ordinates as Figure 39A. Points ● show a further stage of recovery at 360 sec. to 430 sec. after the passage of the depolarizing current. The broken line shows the curve of Figure 39A, which was obtained for this motoneurone both before the depolarizing current and after complete recovery at 510 sec. to 580 sec. Note that compared with Figure 39A the ordinate scale is halved relative to the abscissal scale. Arrows pointing to each curve indicate respective resting potentials. *B.* As in *A,* but for antidromic inhibitory potentials that are partly illustrated in Figure 38H–L and M–Q. The broken line shows curve of Figure 39B, but at half the ordinate scale as in Figure 44A. *C.* Same motoneurone and IPSP's as in *A,* but showing recovery after the passage of a much longer depolarizing current (5 x 10⁻⁸A for 300 sec.). The curve through the × points is the control curve before the current with the arrow showing resting potential of -67 mV, while immediately after the current (5 sec. to 60 sec.) the curve indicated by ▲ points was obtained. Progressive recovery is shown by the successive groups of records at 120-180 (■),

and 38H–L, the E_{IPSP} is found to be about -35 mV just after the passage of the current (crosses in Figure 44A,B). About 200 sec. later, however, recovery was far advanced, as shown by the series of Figures 37M–Q and 38M–Q, the resting membrane potential being -70 mV, and the E_{IPSP} -66 mV (open circles in Figure 44A,B). Finally, after 9 minutes the resting potential was -74 mV and the E_{IPSP} -80 mV, i.e., recovery was then complete, as may be seen in Figure 39A,B, where the plotted values before the injection (filled circles) and some nine minutes after (open circles) are seen to lie on the same curves.

If the same current was passed through a microelectrode filled with K_2SO_4 solution, there was subsequently a much smaller and more transient displacement of the IPSP toward a depolarizing response, recovery usually being complete within 60 sec. (Figure 45B). Finally, if the current was passed through a tetramethylammonium sulphate electrode, there was subsequently the same change in the IPSP as with a Na_2SO_4 electrode, but recovery was at best slow and incomplete. For example, in Figure 45A the E_{IPSP} was changed from an initial value of -81 mV to -74 mV, -57 mV, and -38 mV by three successive currents of 5×10^{-8}A for 60 sec.

When similarly investigating the after-hyperpolarization by injection of cations, it was argued that its diminution or even reversal could not have been caused by the increase in intracellular concentration of Na^+ or $(CH_3)_4N^+$ ions, but was satisfactorily explained by the concurrent

---

240-300 (+), 420-480 (○), 600-660 (●) and 840-890 (◆) sec, respectively. Note that as shown by the arrows the resting potential had increased at 14 min. to 15 min. to a value (-84 mV) considerably in excess of the initial value (-67 mV). *D*. Plot of recovery after depolarizing currents of responses of *A* and *C*. Zero on abscissal time scale gives instant of cessation of the current, the points to the left thereof giving the initial control values before the currents of 90 sec. and 300 sec. duration (note scale readings of -90 sec. and -300 sec.). Points indicated by ▲ and ■ plot, respectively, the equilibrium potentials and the resting potentials for the series of *A* after a 90-sec. current, while ○ and ● give the corresponding values for the series of *C* after a 300-sec. current (Coombs, Eccles, and Fatt, 1955b).

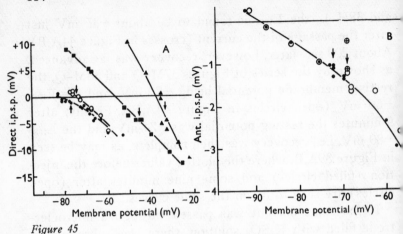

Figure 45

A. A double microelectrode filled with 1.6 M-tetramethylammonium sulphate was inserted into a biceps-semitendinosus motoneurone. Points shown as ● plot direct IPSP against membrane potential as in Figure 39A. After a depolarizing current of 3×10^{-8}A for 60 sec., the points are shown as ○, while points ■ give records after a repetition of this current and ▲ after a still further repetition. Arrows indicate mean resting potentials for each curve. *B.* A double microelectrode filled with 0.6 M-K_2SO_4 was inserted into an unidentified motoneurone. Points shown as ● plot antidromic IPSP against membrane potential as in Figure 39B. After a depolarizing current of 10×10^{-8}A for 90 sec. the records are plotted as ○. The two records immediately following the current are shown by ⊕, the first being high above the control curve and the second showing a considerable recovery at about 15 sec. Arrows marking the resting potentials show that it was depressed by about 3 mV after the current (Coombs, Eccles, and Fatt, 1955b).

depletion of intracellular K^+ ions, if the after-hyperpolarization was caused specifically by the movement of these latter ions. With the IPSP the interpretation of such experiments is complicated by the changes in intracellular chloride, which must be increased by the inward passage of Cl^- ions that will be carrying a considerable fraction of the applied current from the interior of the neurone outward across the surface membrane (Coombs *et al.*, 1955b). The consequent increase in intracellular Cl^- ion concentration would itself tend to displace the IPSP in the depolarizing direction (cf. Figure 40), whereas it would have no effect on the after-hyperpolarization, which is produced only by the movement of K$^+$ ions. The small and transient change produced in the IPSP by the passage of the current through a K$_2$SO$_4$-filled electrode (Figure 45B) provides a control of the effect attributable to this influx of Cl$^-$ ions across the surface membrane.

It must be remembered, however, that the control is imperfect since it only can be applied to a different neurone, and, moreover, as the current through a Na$_2$SO$_4$- or [(CH$_3$)$_4$N]$_2$SO$_4$-filled electrode causes progressive depletion of intracellular K$^+$ ions, a progressively larger proportion will be carried across the membrane by the inward movement of Cl$^-$ ions. Hence, the increase in intracellular Cl$^-$ concentration would be expected to be larger than with the control observations in which the current was applied through a K$_2$SO$_4$-filled electrode (cf. Coombs *et al.*, 1955b). Nevertheless, the time course of recovery from dosage with Cl$^-$ ions is so much faster (time constant about 30 sec.) than the recovery observed in Figure 44A,B (time constant about 200 sec.) that most of the diminution in the E$_{IPSP}$ must have been due to some change other than the increase in intracellular Cl$^-$ ion concentration.

It seems that the only possible explanation must be based on the depletion of intracellular K$^+$ ions, which is effective in diminishing the E$_{IPSP}$ because the net movement of K$^+$ ions across the subsynaptic membrane contributes to the generation of the IPSP. It already has been shown that the equilibrium potential for K$^+$ ions (E$_K$) is normally at about -90 mV, i.e., at 20 mV more hyperpolarization than the resting potential; hence a hyperpolarizing potential would be produced if activated inhibitory synapses increased the permeability of the subsynaptic membrane to K$^+$ ions. With depletion of intracellular potassium there would be a lowering of the E$_K$ even below the resting membrane potential, hence it is possible to explain the conversion of the IPSP to a depolarizing response as in Figures 37K and 38K. Recovery would occur as the intracellular K$^+$ ion concentration is restored by diffusion and by the operation of a potassium pump, as has already been discussed. It is to be noted that, subsequent to potassium depletion, the time course of recovery toward the initial hyperpolarizing response follows much the same time course for the after-hyperpolarization and for the IPSP, the time constant being about 200 sec. after a moderate K^+ ion depletion (cf. filled triangles of Figure 44D). After more severe K^+ ion depletion there is a slower recovery, as illustrated by the successive plotted series of Figure 44C and the open circles of Figure 44D.

4. The Ionic Mechanism
Responsible for Generating the IPSP

Reference to Table 2 shows that all those ions which have been found to be effective in modifying the IPSP are, in the hydrated state, smaller than a certain critical size, but may be anions or cations. In order to be effective, these ions must move freely through the subsynaptic membrane under activated inhibitory synapses, while all larger ions are virtually ineffective because they are excluded or

TABLE 2. *Ion diameters in aqueous solution as derived from limiting ion conductances and expressed relative to $K^+ = 1.00$*

Values derived from Landolt-Börnstein (1936)

The horizontal broken line gives the division between the small ions that pass readily through the subsynaptic inhibitory membrane and the larger ions that pass with much greater difficulty or not at all.

Cations		Anions	
K^+	1.00	Br^-	0.9
		Cl^-	0.9
		NO_3^-	1.0
		SCN^-	1.1
Na$^+$	1.47	HCO_3^-	1.6
$N(CH_3)_4^+$	1.60	$CH_3CO_2^-$	1.8
		SO_4^{2-}	1.8
		$H_2PO_4^-$	2.0
		HPO_4^{2-}	2.5

admitted much less freely. These observations are readily explained by assuming that the inhibitory transmitter substance causes the subsynaptic membrane to become a sieve whose pores admit the passage both of anions and cations as large as the SCN^- ion, regardless of charge, while all larger ions pass with great difficulty or not at all. In particular, the Na^+ ion must be very effectively excluded, else the IPSP would not be a hyperpolarizing response. This attractive postulate requires further testing, particularly by ions having a diameter in the critical range between SCN^- and Na^+ ions. It has been found that the four species of small anions, Cl^-, NO^-_3, Br^-, and SCN^-, are about equally effective in modifying the IPSP; hence, in view of the apparent absence of any modifying influence due to charge, it seems justifiable to assume that the other ion species which determines the IPSP, the K^+ ion, has a similar mobility across the subsynaptic membrane, for its diameter is similar to that of the effective anions (cf. Table 2).

Though the intracellular injections of several other anion species were as effective as Cl^- ions in diminishing the E_{IPSP}, their negligible concentration must make them normally ineffective; hence it appears that the movements across the subsynaptic membrane of only Cl^- and K^+ ions ordinarily contribute significantly to the production of the IPSP. Their relative roles can be assessed by consideration of the various equilibrium potentials. Reference must be made to the original paper for a more rigorous treatment (Coombs *et al.*, 1955b, pp. 360-62). If it is assumed that the inhibitory transmitter makes the subsynaptic membrane equally permeable to K^+ and Cl^- ions, the E_{IPSP} should be approximately midway between E_K and E_{Cl}. Thus with $E_{IPSP} = -80$ mV, and $E_K = -90$ mV, E_{Cl} will equal -70 mV, which is approximately the resting membrane potential, i.e., it appears that the chloride ions are normally in diffusional equilibrium across the neuronal membrane. This inference is in agreement with investigations on the membranes of giant axons of muscle fibres and of erythrocytes (cf. Hodgkin, 1951; Davson, 1952). If Cl⁻ ions are thus in diffusional equilibrium at the resting membrane potential, during the production of the IPSP the movements of K^+ and Cl^- ions across the subsynaptic membranes will have opposing actions, the net movement of K^+ ions giving hyperpolarization, while the net movement of Cl^- ions will act to diminish the amount of hyperpolarization so produced. It must not be concluded, however, that the movement of Cl^- ions has no inhibitory function. It is evident that, when it is effective, inhibition must be exerted against a synaptic depolarization which alone is large enough to generate impulses. Under such conditions, the membrane potential will be 10 mV or more below the resting potential and the value for E_{Cl}. Consequently, the net movement of the Cl^- ions across the subsynaptic membrane will aid the K^+ ions in diminishing the depolarization and so be effective in inhibiting the reflex discharge of impulses (cf. Chapter IV).

It should be pointed out that the experimental evidence which indicates that the K^+ ion movement across the subsynaptic membrane contributes to the production of the IPSP is less convincing than the evidence for the contribution from anion movement. The participation of K^+ ions, however, is further indicated by the evidence that the movements of K^+ ions contribute to two other types of inhibitory potentials: that given by crustacean muscle (Fatt and Katz, 1953), and that produced by acetylcholine in cardiac muscle (Burgen and Terroux, 1953).

Reasons already have been given for assuming that the IPSP produced by direct inhibitory action has virtually the same time course as that produced by a single impulse at an inhibitory synapse. As derived in this way, the unitary time course would have a rising phase lasting about 1.5 msec., and after 2 msec. it would decay exponentially with a time constant of about 3 msec. As shown in Figure 36A this time course is produced by the action on the postsynaptic membrane (time constant about 2.5 msec.) of a subsynaptic current that has a brief initial peak and rapidly declines to a low residuum. Thus a single inhibitory impulse would cause the subsynaptic membrane to develop the characteristic ionic permeability at a high level for less than 2 msec. The consequent flux of K⁺ and Cl⁻ ions along their electrochemical gradients produces the potential change which the intracellular electrode records from the whole postsynaptic membrane.

In a diagrammatic representation (Figure 46A) of the

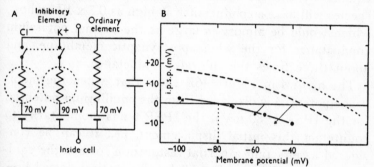

Figure 46

A. Diagrammatic representation of the electrical properties of an ordinary element of the neuronal membrane and of an inhibitory element with K⁺ and Cl⁻ ion components in parallel. Further description in text. *B.* IPSP/membrane potential curves drawn on co-ordinates having equal values as described in the text. The arrows give the actual potential loci for IPSP responses corresponding to the four filled circles on the `continuous line, i.e., the IPSP starts at the base of the arrow and reaches its summit at the apex of the arrow (Coombs, Eccles, and Fatt, 1955b).

electrical properties of the inhibitory subsynaptic membrane and the postsynaptic membrane in general, we can envisage the inhibitory transmitter as operating a ganged switch (shown by dotted line) which turns on current through the potassium and chloride components of the inhibitory elements. It is to be understood, of course, that these components do not occupy different holes in the sieve-like membrane. They are merely drawn separately for diagrammatic convenience. The potassium and chloride equilibrium potentials are shown as −90 mV and −70 mV respectively.

The steepest slope observed for a direct IPSP at a normal membrane potential has been about 5V per sec. This charging rate of the membrane capacity (3×10^{-9}F) indicates that the inhibitory current through the subsynaptic membrane may be as large as 1.5×10^{-8}A. Since the potential driving this current is only 10 mV, the conductance through the direct inhibitory subsynaptic areas may be as high as 1.5×10^{-6} mhos. If this conductance is shared equally by the K^+ and Cl^- ionic mechanisms, each ion species will have a conductance as high as 0.7×10^{-6} mhos., which would be almost as large as the normal potassium conductance for the whole postsynaptic membrane, and about three times the chloride conductance.

The arrows in Figure 46B show that, when the membrane potential is displaced from the equilibrium potential for the IPSP (-80 mV), the IPSP tends momentarily to counteract this initial displacement, i.e., it can be considered as effecting a partial restoration toward the equilibrium potential as indicated by the vertical dotted line. With small displacements this relative restoration was only 16 per cent in Figure 46B. Values as high as 60 per cent have been observed for the restoration when the ionic composition of the motoneurone was altered so that there was an increased ionic flux across the subsynaptic membrane, as is shown in the curves to the right in Figure 45A, and the curves shown by broken lines in Figure 46B.

5. The Ionic Interchange
between a Motoneurone and Its Environment

This section properly belongs to Chapter I, but it is so dependent on the investigations of Chapters II and III that it is considered more conveniently here. Since the interchange of Cl^- ions may be presumed to be purely diffusional, it is treated appropriately before the more complex processes governing the Na^+ and K^+ ion exchanges.

a. The diffusional exchange of Cl⁻ ions

Since all measurements have to be made with an intra-cellular electrode filled with a chloride salt, it is necessary to consider the initial conditions that obtain when such an electrode is inserted into a motoneurone. In order to avoid complications arising from changes in the cation content of the motoneurone, it is important to have the electrode filled with a potassium salt, i.e., a KCl-filled electrode is required. Actually, identical behaviour is observed with KNO_3-, KBr-, and KSCN-filled electrodes (cf. Figures 40, 41, and 42), indicating that for present purposes the respective anions are equivalent to Cl⁻ ions.

We already have observed that the IPSP changes toward a depolarizing response shortly after insertion of such microelectrodes into a motoneurone (Figures 40 and 41), an effect which was attributed to the increased intracellular concentration which is produced by diffusion out of the microelectrode of the Cl⁻ (or equivalent anion). A further temporary change in the same direction is observed after an injection of the anion species has been brought about electrophoretically by means of a current that crosses the neuronal membrane in a hyperpolarizing direction (Figures 40, 41, and 42). If the current is passed in the opposite direction, i.e., a depolarizing current, there is subsequently the opposite change in the IPSP, which is even temporarily converted into a hyperpolarizing response (Figure 47B), but the effect is always transient (Figure 47C–F). Recovery to the initial depolarizing response occurs in an approximately exponential manner with a time constant that does not differ significantly from that observed for recovery from the opposite displacement (Figure 47I). Presumably the temporary phase of hyperpolarizing IPSP is indicative of a decrease in concentration of the effective anions. This decrease would be consequential on the suppression which the applied current produces in the diffusion of anions out of the electrode. Under such conditions diffusional exchange across the surface

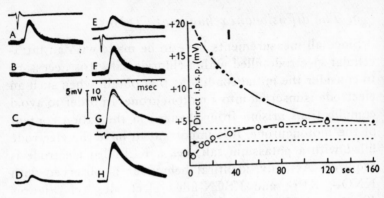

Figure 47

A–H. A single microelectrode filled with 3 M-KNO₃ was inserted into a biceps-semitendinosus motoneurone. *A* shows the depolarizing IPSP set up by a quadriceps group Ia volley. After the passage of a depolarizing current (4 x 10⁻⁸A for 90 sec.) there was a momentary reversal of the IPSP to the hyperpolarizing type, *B*, followed by recovery to the original response, *C–F*. *G* and *H* show EPSP's set up by monosynaptic excitation before and immediately after the same depolarizing current. Records of the quadriceps afferent volley in L6 dorsal root are shown in *A* and *F*, while the biceps-semitendinosus afferent volley similarly recorded is seen between *G* and *H*. The resting potential was −79 mV before passage of current and −82 mV immediately after. Potential scale gives 5 mV for records *A* and *F*, and 10 mV for *G* and *H*. Time scale applies to all records. *I*. Open circles plot recovery of IPSP's for series partly illustrated in *B–F*, the initial depolarizing IPSP (Figure 47A) being shown by the open circle on the broken line, which thus represents a base line. Time is measured from cessation of current. Filled circles represent recovery series for the IPSP after the earlier passage of a hyperpolarizing current (3 x 10⁻⁸A for 90 sec.), the initial value for the IPSP again having a base line drawn through it (cf. Figure 42) (Coombs, Eccles, and Fatt, 1955b).

membrane would cause the Cl⁻ concentration to approach the level that normally exists in the motoneurone.

Conceivably these various changes in the IPSP might have been brought about by changes which the applied current would produce in the distribution of anions within the motoneurone, for the IPSP merely signals the relative concentration of anions across the inhibitory subsynaptic membrane. However, on the assumption that the mobility of ions is not significantly depressed within the neurone (cf. Hodgkin and Keynes, 1953; Caldwell, 1955), it can be shown that, for a structure having the dimensions of a motoneurone, virtual uniformity of ionic distribution will be re-established within one second of the cessation of the applied current (Coombs et al., 1955b). By making a series of probable assumptions, such as uniformity of the electric potential field across the membrane and equality of K^+ and Cl^- ion permeabilities across the inhibitory sub-synaptic membrane, an equation has been derived (cf. Goldman, 1943; Hodgkin and Katz, 1949) which relates the slope of the rising phase of the IPSP to the membrane potential and the concentrations of K^+ and Cl^- ions on the two sides of the membrane (cf. equation 9, Coombs et al., 1955b). If a probable value is assumed for the internal concentration of Cl^- ions (plus any other effective anion) at the end of the applied current, it is possible to calculate the subsequent time course of this concentration if given the maximum slopes of the rising phases of the IPSP's at a series of intervals thereafter. Actually, the curves of Figure 47I are not significantly different, if the maximum slopes of the IPSP's are plotted instead of their summits. Furthermore, the calculated concentrations for the internal anions follow curves that decay exponentially with time constants almost identical with those of Figure 47I.

It can be concluded that, after an applied current has caused either an increase or decrease in the intracellular concentration of Cl^-, NO_3^-, or Br^- ions, the time course of restoration of the initial concentration is approximately exponential. Because of the high ionic concentration in the microelectrode, there would be, in the absence of current, a steady output of anions (and cations) by diffusion. The initial steady-state condition would be restored as the net outward anionic flux across the surface membrane falls or rises to equal the output from the electrode. Thus, it would be expected that the time constant of recovery, whose mean value is about 30 sec. (derived from the mean half-time of about 20 sec.), is dependent on the properties of the neurone and not of the electrode, and that it would be approximately the same in both directions, as is actually observed (Figure 47I).

The conditions may be represented diagrammatically as in Figure 48, where C_i represents the concentration of

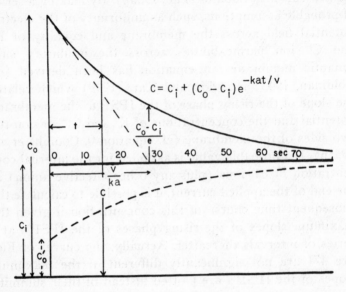

Figure 48

The exponentially decaying curves plot the time courses of the intracellular concentration of effective anions according to the theoretical treatment developed in the text. For the upper curve at any time, t, the total concentration of Cl^- plus NO_3^- ions, C, is given by the equation $C = C_1 + (C_o - C_1)e^{-kat/v}$, as described in the text. The lower curve plotted as the broken line is similarly defined, C'_o being the initial concentration.

Cl^- ions after diffusional equilibrium had been established between the microelectrode and the motoneurone. Under such conditions, there would be a steady diffusional efflux of Cl^- ions from the high concentration within the microelectrode, and an equivalent net efflux across the surface membrane of the motoneurone. It has been shown (Coombs *et al.*, 1955b) that the rate of diffusion of Cl^- ions from the microelectrode would have the order of magnitude that is required to account for the observed changes in the IPSP. A hyperpolarizing current would increase greatly the efflux of Cl⁻ ions out of the microelectrode, there being on termination of the current an increased value for $(Cl^-)_{int}$, which is shown in Figure 48 by C_o. As a consequence, the outward diffusion is much greater than the inward diffusion of Cl⁻ ions, the initial value of C_i being attained by an exponential decay. This is given approximately by the equation (cf. Coombs *et al.*, 1955b)

$$C = C_i + (C_o - C_i) e^{-kat/v},$$

where C is the value of $(Cl^-)_{int}$ at time t after cessation of the current, a and v are respectively the effective surface area and volume of the motoneurone, and k is the proportionality constant that at the resting membrane potential relates the ionic flux across its membrane to the intracellular concentration, C. The small alterations produced in k by the small changes in the membrane potential (cf. Figure 47) have been neglected. The time constant of the exponential decay, $\frac{v}{ka}$, is approximately 30 sec. As is actually observed (Figure 47I), approximately the same time constant would be expected for recovery from the depletion of Cl⁻ ion concentration that is brought about by a depolarizing current (cf. broken line, Figure 48).

Having determined the value for $\frac{v}{ka}$, it is possible to calculate the total Cl⁻ ion efflux from a motoneurone under normal steady-state conditions. Thus, if M_{Cl} denotes the outward flux of Cl⁻ ions, the total efflux will be given by two expressions, which may therefore be equated:

$$aM_{Cl} = -ka \, (Cl)_{int},$$

where $(Cl)_{int}$ is the normal intracellular concentration of Cl⁻ ions. Since, at the resting membrane potential, the time constant, v/ka, has been found to be about 30 sec. for Cl⁻ ions,

$$aM_{Cl} = \frac{-v(Cl)_{int}}{30} = -0.07 \text{ p. mole sec.}^{-1}$$

if $(Cl)_{int} = 9$ mM (p. 24) and $v = 2.5 \times 10^{-7}$ cm³. Since this chloride efflux of 0.07 p. mole sec.⁻¹ occurs at the normal steady state, and since it has not been necessary to postulate a chloride pump, there will be the same diffusional influx. It thus is possible to calculate the membrane conductance for chloride ions, G_{Cl}, from the formula derived by Hodgkin (1951).

$$G_{Cl} = \frac{F^2}{RT} M_{Cl},$$

where F, R, and T have the usual connotation. The value so calculated for aG_{Cl}, 0.25×10^{-6} mho., represents the chloride conductance for the effective surface area of a standard motoneurone, and hence is to be compared with the approximate measured value, 1.2×10^{-6} mho., for the total conductance. This proportion of approximately 20 per cent to 30 per cent of the total membrane conductance is in good agreement with the proportions calculated for the chloride conductance of giant axons and striated muscle fibres (Hodgkin and Katz, 1949; Hodgkin, 1951; Hodgkin and Huxley, 1952b; Shanes, Grundfest, and Freygang, 1953). The most unreliable estimate used in the above calculation was the value for the volume of the motoneurone. It has been suggested that this estimate could be too low by a factor of two (Coombs et al., 1955a). By assuming double the value for v, G_{Cl} is doubled in size and so would account for almost half of the total conductance. If an area of 5×10^{-4} cm^2 is assumed for a, i.e., for the effective surface area of the motoneurone, a value of 0.07 p. mole sec.$^{-1}$ for this surface corresponds to a value for M_{Cl} of 140 p. mole cm^{-2} sec.$^{-1}$, which is several times greater than the largest ionic fluxes observed for giant axons or muscle fibres in the resting state (cf. Hodgkin, 1951; Shanes and Berman, 1955).

b. The interchange of Na+ and K+ ions across the surface membrane of a motoneurone

When the K+ ions of a motoneurone have been partly replaced by Na+ ions, it has been seen that large changes occurred in both the rising and falling phases of the spike potential (Figure 26A), in the after-hyperpolarization, (Figure 26B,C) and in the IPSP (Figures 37, 38). Recovery from all these changes was observed to occur with approximately the same time courses (cf. Figure 44D). On the other hand, if $(CH_3)_4 N^+$ ions were substituted for the K^+ ions, similar changes were observed (cf. Figures 27, 45A) except for the rising phase of the spike, but at best recovery was slow and incomplete. It appears, therefore, that, as with giant axons (Hodgkin and Keynes, 1955), there is coupling of the outward sodium pump with the inward potassium pump so that the K^+ ion concentration cannot be restored if there is not an equivalent amount of Na^+ ions to be pumped outward. Probably also, as suggested for giant axons (Hodgkin and Keynes, 1955), the activity of the pump is controlled by the internal concentration of Na^+ ions.

The recovery of the K^+ ion concentration is indicated much more effectively by the experimental data, in particular by the after-hyperpolarization (cf. Figure 26B,C) and by the IPSP (cf. Figure 44D), and presumably it may be used to give an approximate measure of the activity of the coupled sodium-potassium pump. When about 25 p. mole of Na^+ ions was added in substitution for the loss of about 20 p. mole of K^+ ions and the gain of about 5 p. mole of Cl^- ions, recovery was more than half complete in about 150 sec. Thus Na^+ ions were being extruded by the pump at the rate of about 1 p. mole in 6 sec. If the area of the surface membrane of the motoneurone is 5×10^{-4} cm^2, the rate of pumping is 300 p. mole cm^{-2} sec.$^{-1}$, which is about 6 times faster than the maximum rate found for giant axons (Hodgkin and Keynes, 1955; Shanes and Berman, 1955). This difference would be largely explicable by the higher temperature of the motoneurone (38°C as against 18°C), which would cause metabolism to be several times higher. There is considerable uncertainty, however, in the calculated rate for motoneurones, particularly in the assessment of the effective surface area.

B. INHIBITORY RESPONSES OF
CRUSTACEAN STRETCH RECEPTOR CELLS

The dendritic terminals of a crustacean stretch receptor cell are closely invested by the synaptic terminals of a single inhibitory fibre (Figure 49A; Alexandrowicz, 1951; 1952; Florey and Florey, 1955). It has been possible to record intracellularly the responses produced in the stretch receptor cell by single impulses in the inhibitory fibre (Kuffler and Eyzaguirre, 1955). As shown in Figure 49B, trains of five impulses at 20 per sec. produced very different effects according to the level at which the membrane potential was set by stretching the attached muscle. For example, with a membrane depolarization of 16.5 mV in the left record of B, the inhibitory impulses caused a peak repolarization of 9.7 mV, while progressive decrease of the membrane depolarization caused diminution and then reversal of the inhibitory responses. The equilibrium potential so determined for the inhibitory response is shown by the broken line at a membrane depolarization of 6.7 mV. Figure 49B is remarkable in that it shows an inhibitory response that compensates for as much as 90 per cent of the initial displacement of membrane potential. With the direct IPSP of motoneurones the compensation is normally only about 20 per cent (cf. Figure 46B), while with inhibitory action on crustacean muscle, compensation is below 10 per cent (Fatt and Katz, 1953).

The equilibrium potential for the inhibitory response of the receptor cell was, as in Figure 49B, invariably on the depolarized side of the membrane potential obtaining in the unstretched state. Usually it was only a few millivolts of depolarization, but sometimes it was much further removed, even so far that the IPSP produced a depolarization sufficient to generate an impulse, just as was observed with the IPSP of motoneurones injected with Cl^- or NO_3^- ions (cf. Figures 40, 41).

With the crustacean stretch receptor, the displacement of the equilibrium potential for the IPSP in the depolariz-

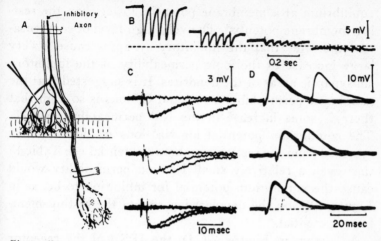

Figure 49

A. Diagrammatic illustration of the arrangement of slow and fast adapting cells in the stretch receptor organs of the eighth thoracic segment of crayfish. The inhibitory axon (black solid line) branches and innervates both receptor cells at the regions where the dendritic terminals are in contact with the muscle fibres of the receptor organs. The microelectrode is drawn as inserted into the "slow" cell. If the I axon is stimulated by the lower pair of electrodes the inhibitory impulse will reach the dendritic terminals of the slow cell by an axon reflex. *B.* Effect of repetitive I impulses at four different membrane potential levels, as shown by the respective base line levels, which were set by graded stretch of the receptor organ. The broken line indicates approximately the equilibrium potential for the inhibitory postsynaptic potentials, IPSP's, which reversed to depolarizing responses when the membrane potential was below this level. *C, D.* Superimposed IPSP's evoked in each case by single and by double inhibitory impulses at various intervals (18 msec., 6 msec. and 2 msec. in *C*). The receptor organ in *C* is under light stretch, while in *D* it is relaxed, hence the respective hyperpolarizing and depolarizing IPSP's (Kuffler and Eyzaguirre, 1955).

ing direction could not be attributed to Cl⁻ diffusion from the microelectrode, and depolarizing IPSP's were even observed by extracellular recording (Kuffler and Eyzaguirre, 1955). Electrophoretic injections of ions have not yet been attempted with the crustacean receptor cell, so only tentative explanations may be offered. It seems unlikely that an inhibitory ionic mechanism involving the movement of K⁺ and Cl⁻ ions would normally have an equilibrium at a membrane potential lower than the resting membrane potential. The very high level of compensation indicates that the inhibitory synapses cause a very large increase in the ionic permeability of the inhibitory subsynaptic areas of the dendrites. It is suggested that the membrane permeability to K^+ and Cl^- ions is so high that there is some increase in the Na^+ permeability as well. The equilibrium potential for Na^+ ions would be so far removed from the resting membrane potential (cf. Table 1) that even a relatively small Na^+ ion permeability would cause the equilibrium potential for inhibition to be, as in Figure 49B, on the depolarizing side of the resting membrane potential.

As shown in Figure 49C,D, the IPSP of the receptor cell has approximately the same time course whether it is of the repolarizing or depolarizing type. It rises to a summit in 2 msec. to 3 msec. and thereafter declines approximately exponentially with a time constant of 15 msec. to 20 msec. Figure 49C,D also shows that a second inhibitory impulse is unable by summation to produce an IPSP which is larger than the initial response. The apparent ceiling in the level of the IPSP is correlated with the high level of compensation (cf. Figure 49B). Repetitive inhibitory impulses were able to build up an increased IPSP when the compensation was lower.

There is evidence that the receptor cell IPSP differs from that of the motoneurone in that the active inhibitory effect continues at a high level throughout the whole duration of the IPSP. The long duration of the active inhibitory effect is indicated by the following observations. (1) The size of the antidromic spike potential of the receptor cell is depressed during the full duration of the IPSP (Kuffler and Eyzaguirre, Figure 14), which indicates that there is a continued high conductance of the subsynaptic inhibitory areas for at least 20 msec. (2) The potential generated by a blocked antidromic response has a smaller size and faster time course for as long as 20 msec. after the onset of the IPSP (Kuffler and Eyzaguirre, Figure 15), which again indicates a continued high conductance of the inhibitory areas. (3) Repetitive inhibitory volleys are followed by a prolonged (more than 200 msec.) potential, which seems attributable to an accumulation of the inhibitory transmitter substance (Kuffler and Eyzaguirre, Figure 8).

The after-hyperpolarization which follows a motoneurone spike has an equilibrium potential at about −90 mV, which is significantly different from that of the IPSP at −80 mV. Similarly, the after-potential that follows the spike response of a crustacean receptor cell (Figure 33A,B) has been shown to have a different equilibrium potential from the IPSP, which may be either higher or lower (Kuffler and Eyzaguirre, Figures 10, 11). The interaction of the after-potential with the IPSP has provided further evidence that the conductance of the subsynaptic inhibitory areas is so high that a superimposed after-potential is virtually ineffective in causing any change in the IPSP (Kuffler and Eyzaguirre, Figure 12).

C. POSSIBLE INHIBITORY RESPONSES OF SYMPATHETIC GANGLION CELLS

Laporte and Lorente de Nó (1950) found that, when the superior cervical ganglion of the turtle was deeply curarized so that the EPSP was virtually eliminated, a presynaptic volley still set up a large and prolonged postsynaptic hyperpolarization, which was propagated electrotonically along the postganglionic trunk. Evidently this hyperpolarization was a response of nerve cells that was directly evoked by presynaptic impulses. Presumably it was normally present and was uncovered by the specific depression of the excitatory responses by tubocurarine. This hyperpolarizing response, or P wave, also was observed when the excitatory responses of the superior cervical ganglion of the rabbit were depressed by curarizing agents and anticholinesterases (R. M. Eccles, 1952b).

It seems that this hyperpolarizing response must be regarded as an example of synaptic inhibitory action as defined at the beginning of this chapter. It has not yet been established, however, that there are preganglionic impulses having a special inhibitory function, and that physiologically they have an effective inhibitory action (cf. Eccles, 1936a; Lorente de Nó and Laporte, 1950; Job and Lundberg, 1953). There is evidence that a special synaptic mechanism giving P waves may not be present with some ganglia. A possible suggestion is that adrenaline and noradrenaline could be the synaptic transmitter substances concerned in setting up the P wave, for they exert a powerful depressant action on ganglion cells (Marrazzi, 1939; Lundberg, 1952). Adrenaline, however, has been found to cause the depression while producing little or no hyperpolarization (Lundberg, 1952), hence it seems unlikely that it could be the transmitter generating the P wave.

D. SUMMARY

It appears that inhibitory action on a nerve cell is brought about by a depression of the EPSP below the threshold level for initiation of an impulse. This is effected by a specific increase in ionic conductance and the consequent change in membrane potential, the IPSP, which may be a hyperpolarization of the resting membrane, as in the motoneurone, or even a small depolarization, as in the crustacean stretch receptor cell. An intermediate type of inhibitory action occurs on crustacean muscle, where no potential is generated at the resting membrane potential, i.e., the inhibitory ionic mechanism is in equilibrium at this potential. There is no evidence that inhibitory action on nerve cells is in part due to a curare-like action of the inhibitory transmitter, such as has been demonstrated for crustacean neuromuscular transmission (Fatt and Katz, 1953; Fatt, 1954).

With motoneurones the IPSP set up by a single synchronous activation of inhibitory synapses runs a time course which is approximately a mirror image of the EPSP, though it has a longer latency and a faster decay. It is produced by a subsynaptic current that reaches its maximum within 1 msec. and rapidly declines therefrom, there being little or no residual current after 2 msec. It is necessary to postulate that a specific transmitter substance causes the inhibitory synaptic response of the motoneurone by changing the ionic permeability of the subsynaptic membrane. It has been shown that the membrane becomes highly permeable to Cl^- and K^+ ions, while retaining a high degree of impermeability to Na^+ ions. The equilibrium potential for the IPSP, about -80 mV, is a compromise between the equilibrium potentials of about -90 mV and -70 mV for the K^+ and Cl^- ions respectively. The subsynaptic membrane also shows the same permeability change to other small ions, Br^-, NO^-_3, and SCN^-.

With crustacean muscle it seems that a similar mechanism is responsible for inhibition, though only the role of K^+ ion permeability has so far been established (Fatt and Katz, 1953). The inhibitory ionic mechanism for crustacean stretch receptor cells has not yet been investigated in detail, but there is evidence that the specific ionic permeability generating the IPSP continues throughout the greater part of the duration of the IPSP. It is suggested that the membrane permeability to K^+ and Cl^- ions becomes so high that even some Na^+ ions are admitted. As a consequence, the equilibrium potential for the IPSP is actually at a low level of depolarization.

CHAPTER IV

THE INTERACTION OF THE EXCITATORY AND INHIBITORY RESPONSES OF NERVE CELLS

A. MOTONEURONES

In the preceding chapter an account was given of the postsynaptic events that were produced by inhibitory synaptic activity. It was shown that there was a great increase in the permeability to some ions, notably K^+ and Cl^-, and that as a consequence electric currents flowed across the subsynaptic inhibitory membrane causing a change in the potential across the postsynaptic membrane as a whole, which has been called the IPSP. The present problem is to show how these inhibitory currents and the IPSP generated thereby cause the suppression of reflex discharge, which is the overt sign of central inhibitory action. Particular attention will be paid to the direct inhibitory action on testing monosynaptic reflex discharges, because under these conditions the inhibitory action on reflexes has been studied most precisely (Lloyd, 1946; Laporte and Lloyd, 1952; Bradley, Easton, and Eccles, 1953).

1. The Inhibitory Curve for Direct Inhibition

In the standard technique the testing monosynaptic reflex has been set up at various intervals after the volley exerting the direct inhibitory action, i.e., after a volley in the large afferent fibres from the annulo-spiral endings of muscles reciprocally antagonist to those whose motoneurones are under test. At any test interval the depression of the size of the testing monosynaptic reflex gives a measure of the proportion of motoneurones inhibited, and hence it is assumed to measure the intensity of inhibitory action on an average motoneurone. This assumption is justified if the testing reflex occurs in a considerable fraction of the population of motoneurones under investigation, for only under such conditions is there likely to be an approximately linear relationship between these two quantities. It is seen in Figure 50 that the inhibition is first

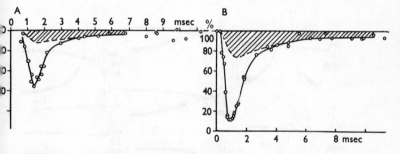

Figure 50

Reproductions of two direct inhibitory curves with the plotted points through which the curves are drawn (Figure 2A, C, Bradley *et al.,* 1953). Ordinates show, for the various test intervals, the mean reflex spikes expressed as percentages of the control value. The broken lines delimit the inhibitory effect which can be attributed simply to the hyperpolarization of the IPSP at its control intensity, and which is distinguished by hatching. There is a large additional inhibitory action at shorter test intervals, which is attributed to the increased subsynaptic currents through the IPSP elements and the consequent potentiation of the IPSP (Coombs, Eccles, and Fatt, 1955d).

observed when the testing excitatory volley enters the spinal cord a fraction of a millisecond after the inhibitory volley, and that thereafter there is a rapid increase to a maximum and a decline therefrom, with eventually a much slower decline with intervals beyond 3 msec. to 4 msec. (cf. Bradley, Easton, and Eccles, 1953).

It has been assumed that the IPSP generated by group Ia afferent impulses is the cause of their direct inhibitory action. Hyperpolarization of the surface membrane would be expected to depress excitability, and the observed hyperpolarization (the IPSP) had a time course bearing some resemblance to the inhibitory curve for direct inhibition. The only serious discrepancy would appear to concern the respective latent periods.

In Figure 51 the inhibitory volley in quadriceps Ia afferent fibres entered the spinal cord at various intervals before the testing excitatory volley in biceps-semitendinosus afferent fibres. When alone, this monosynaptic excitatory volley always evoked the discharge of an impulse by

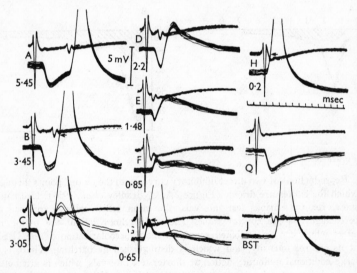

Figure 51

Lower records give intracellular responses evoked in a biceps-semitendinosus motoneurone by group Ia volleys in quadriceps and biceps-semitendinosus nerves at the indicated intervals apart, I and J being the respective control responses. All records are formed by superposition of about twenty faint traces. Potential scale gives 5 mV for intracellular records, upward deflexions indicating membrane depolarization. Upper records are recorded from the L6 dorsal root as in Figure 41. The horizontal arrows mark the approximate potentials at which the spikes are initiated. The low values for these threshold voltages are presumably attributable to depolarization of the motoneurone (cf. Fig. 16B) the resting potential having fallen to -66 mV during this series from an initial value of -72 mV. (Coombs, Eccles, and Fatt, 1955d).

the motoneurone (Figure 51J). Suppression of this discharge was invariably observed with volley intervals lying
within the range of 0.65 msec. to 3.05 msec. (Figure
51D,E,F), while at the extreme values of this range there
was sometimes a failure to inhibit (Figure 51C,G). A

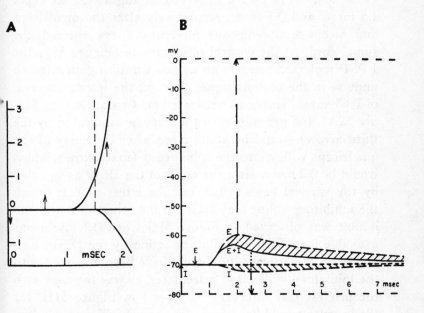

Figure 52

A. Plot of time course of events for the 0.65 msec. test interval of
Fig. 51. The left lower and upper arrows show, respectively, the times of arrival
of the inhibitory and excitatory volleys at the spinal cord. Plotted upwards
is the EPSP, beginning 0.5 msec. after the excitatory volley and rising up
to generate a spike at 0.55 msec. after its onset, as indicated by the arrow.
Plotted downward is the IPSP, beginning 1.5 msec. after the inhibitory
volley, the vertical broken line at this time giving the earliest possible onset
of inhibition. (Coombs, Eccles, and Fatt, 1955d). *B*. Diagrammatic representation of the interaction between a monosynaptic EPSP and a direct
IPSP that is generated during its rising phase, the initial arrows I and E
showing arrival times of the afferent volleys at the spinal cord. The respective equilibrium potentials are 0 mV and −80 mV. Control responses of
IPSP and EPSP are shown by the broken lines labelled I and E, and the
response to the interacting volleys is indicated by the continuous line
(E + I). The arrows drawn from the summits of the I and E potentials
to the respective equilibrium potentials indicate the voltages driving the
subsynaptic currents.

volley interval of 0.65 msec. thus provided the situation giving a measure of the shortest latency for effective inhibitory action on this particular motoneurone.

Figure 52A allows an analysis to be made of the factors concerned in this inhibition at minimum latency. The IPSP and EPSP were observed in Figure 51 to begin 1.5 msec. and 0.5 msec. respectively after the quadriceps and biceps-semitendinosus afferent volleys entered the spinal cord. In the control observations (Figure 51J) the EPSP took 0.55 msec. from its onset until it generated an impulse in the motoneurone. Thus, at the testing interval of 0.65 msec. (interval between first two arrows in Figure 52A), the generation of the impulse (indicated by the third arrow) would be at 1.7 msec. after the entry of the quadriceps volley into the spinal cord (first arrow), which would be 0.2 msec. after the onset of the IPSP as signaled by the vertical broken line, i.e., the latest time at which the inhibitory volley may arrive at the spinal cord and still inhibit was observed in Figure 51G when 0.2 msec. was available for effective inhibitory action by the IPSP. Evidently no inhibitory action could have been expected with the inhibitory volley 0.45 msec. later, as was the case with the briefest test interval (0.2 msec.) in Figure 51H, for the impulse would have been discharged 0.25 msec. before the onset of the IPSP. It is possible, however, that at this test interval inhibition could have occurred in other motoneurones, or even in this motoneurone, when, as a consequence of less strong excitation by the testing volley, it was responding with a longer latent period.

Similar calculations have been made with direct inhibitory action on other motoneurones (cf. J. C. Eccles, 1953, p. 158) and it has always been found that the IPSP is set up early enough to cause the observed inhibition. It may be concluded that, despite its relatively long latency, the IPSP can be effective with the short latency of direct inhibitory action. Thus, it may be assumed that, from sufficiently large populations, one could build up inhibitory curves resembling those of Figure 50.

2. *Interaction between IPSP and EPSP*

Figure 51 further shows that, with superposition of the IPSP and EPSP at various intervals, the generation of an impulse occurred at much the same level of membrane potential, which was about −63 mV, but which must be attained within a critical time. It must not be assumed, however, that the EPSP evoked by the testing volley is simply added on to the conditioning IPSP, and that the inhibitory action is entirely attributable to the hyperpolarization of the IPSP. In Figure 51 a precise study of the interaction between the IPSP and EPSP is not possible because of the spike potential that is generated by the EPSP, both in the control observation and with testing intervals beyond the range of 0.65 msec. to 3.05 msec.

It is important, therefore, to investigate the interaction of the IPSP with the EPSP when uncomplicated by the generation of spikes (Figure 53). The potential records

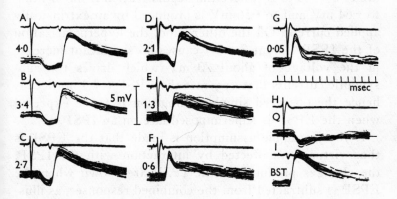

Figure 53

Lower records give, as in Figure 51, intracellular responses (superposition of about 40 faint traces) evoked in a biceps-semitendinosus motoneurone by quadriceps and biceps-semitendinosus volleys which are recorded in the L6 dorsal root (upper records). The volley intervals are marked on each record, being progressively shortened from *A* to *G*. *H* and *I* give control responses to quadriceps and to biceps-semitendinosus volleys alone. Voltage scale gives 5 mV for intracellular recording (Coombs, Eccles, and Fatt, 1955d.)

may be analysed by assuming constancy of either the EPSP or the IPSP and then plotting the change produced in the other as measured by the subtraction technique. Such measurements show that, when superimposed on an EPSP, the IPSP is greatly potentiated, whereas, when an EPSP is superimposed late on an IPSP, there is simple summation of the two potentials. As shown in Figure 52B, this irreciprocity of behaviour is to be expected because of the very different equilibrium potentials for the EPSP and the IPSP. The depolarization of the EPSP significantly displaces the membrane potential from the equilibrium potential for the IPSP, even more than doubling the gap that initially is only about 10 mV. The driving voltage for the subsynaptic currents generating the IPSP would be expected to be correspondingly increased; hence these currents have the greatly increased hyperpolarizing action that is observed. The potentiating effect of depolarization on the IPSP is illustrated in Figure 37D to C to B, where the depolarization from −74 mV to −64 mV and to −56 mV is produced by an extrinsically applied current. On the other hand, the hyperpolarization of the IPSP (about 2 mV) causes no significant increase in the voltage of about 70 mV which drives the subsynaptic currents that generate the EPSP (cf. Figure 22); hence the observed simple summation is to be expected when the EPSP is superimposed late on an IPSP.

If the justifiable assumption is made that the EPSP is thus virtually unaffected by interaction with the IPSP, the changes produced in the IPSP are shown when the EPSP is subtracted from the combined responses, as illustrated in Figure 54A. In the fourth and fifth records the IPSP is almost double in size when its generating current is flowing during the summit of the EPSP. Evidence already has been presented in Chapter III that, with the IPSP set up by direct inhibitory action, the subsynaptic inhibitory current is at a significant intensity for less than 2 msec. (Figure 36A). In that event, it would be expected that appreciable potentiation of the IPSP would occur only when the testing intervals were no longer than 2 msec. to 3 msec., as is actually observed in Figure 54A. At longer intervals (first and second records), the subsynaptic cur-

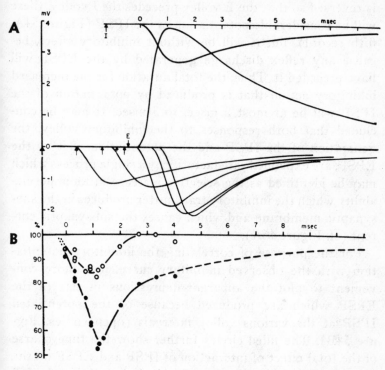

Figure 54

A. The means for five of the records of Figure 53 have been drawn and the control EPSP has been subtracted from the combined response in order to derive the IPSP curves for each interval on the assumption that the EPSP is unaltered (see text). The control IPSP and EPSP curves are plotted above, the arrival of the respective volleys at the cord being signalled by the arrows labelled I and E respectively. The subtracted IPSP curves are shown below, being plotted relative to the control EPSP (see text). *B.* The apparent percentage depression in size of the EPSP (cf. Coombs, Eccles, and Fatt, 1955d, Figure 5A) that is produced on account of the potentiation of the IPSP (cf. Figure 54A) is plotted (open circles) against the respective intervals between the inhibitory and excitatory volleys in the dorsal roots. The actual heights of the EPSP crests in Figure 53 relative to the initial base line are expressed as percentages of the control EPSP in the filled circles. The curve through the filled circles has been extended on the assumption that at the longer intervals unchanged EPSP's are superimposed on the background EPSP (Coombs, Eccles, and Fatt, 1955d).

rents are of negligible intensity before the start of the EPSP; hence there would be very little inhibitory potentiation. Furthermore, if the testing interval is too short, or is reversed so that the E volley precedes the I volley, there will be considerable potentiation of the IPSP (Figure 54A, fifth record), but it will be without inhibitory effect, because any reflex discharge generated by the EPSP will have preceded it. Thus, the total duration for the increased inhibitory action that is produced by potentiation of the IPSP will be at most 2 msec. to 3 msec. It may be concluded that both responses to the inhibitory volley, the generation of the IPSP and the potentiation of it by the EPSP, are explained satisfactorily by a single process which may be identified as the selective increase in ionic permeability which the inhibitory transmitter produces in the subsynaptic membrane and which causes the subsynaptic current (cf. Figure 46A).

For the purpose of correlating the inhibitory potentiation with the observed inhibitory curve, it is more convenient to plot the apparent depressions in size of the EPSP which are produced because of the potentiated IPSP at the various volley intervals (open circles, Figure 54B). The filled circles further show the time course of the total effect of interaction of IPSP and EPSP on the observed depolarization, i.e., the filled circles give the full depressant actions which are exerted on the depolarization of the EPSP by the hyperpolarization of the IPSP, including its potentiated phase.

3. The Correlation of IPSP–EPSP Interaction with the Direct Inhibitory Curve

It has been shown above that by means of two separate actions an inhibitory volley depresses the actual level of depolarization produced by an excitatory volley (filled circles of Figure 54B). A brief action due to the increased subsynaptic currents through the IPSP elements (Figure 54B, open circles) is superimposed on a more prolonged action due to the hyperpolarization of the whole postsynaptic membrane (the IPSP). It is of interest, therefore, that inhibitory curves have been observed to have a configuration indicative of a double composition. For example, the two curves reproduced in Figure 50 have an initial rapid decline merging at about 2 msec. to 3 msec. into a later, approximately exponential decay. The broken line continues this exponential decay further to the left along the time course of an assumed IPSP. Thus, the hatched area would give that component of the inhibitory curve attributable to the hyperpolarization of the IPSP. The remaining component has a duration little longer than 2 msec., having much the same time course as the effective potentiation of the IPSP by the EPSP (Figure 54A,B) and the depression which the IPSP produces in the antidromic spike potential (Figure 36B).

As originally described (Lloyd, 1946), the direct inhibitory curve simply decayed exponentially from its maximum with a time constant of about 4 msec. More recently Laporte and Lloyd (1952) have reported that this simple exponential decay for the direct inhibitory curve was only occasionally observed. Usually there was a rapid decay from the maximum, much as shown in Figure 50. They attributed this deviation to the superposition of a disynaptic excitatory action by group Ib impulses. Curves such as those of Figure 50, however, have been obtained with an afferent volley which could be shown by its spike potential, where it entered the spinal cord, to be restricted to group Ia fibres (cf. Bradley *et al.*, 1953). Further investigation is necessary in order to determine the actual contribution made by the disynaptic excitatory action of group Ib impulses.

It will be observed in Figure 54B that an inhibitory volley appears to exert a considerable depressant action on the EPSP when it is synchronous with the excitatory volley, or even a little later, i.e., to the left of zero. A direct inhibitory action, therefore, might be expected at such intervals, whereas none is observed until the inhibitory volley precedes the excitatory (Figure 50; Laporte and Lloyd, 1952; Bradley *et al.*, 1953). An explanation of this apparent discrepancy is provided by the observation that at such intervals there is depression only of the last part of the rising phase of the EPSP (cf. Figure 53G with Figure 53I), and this part of the EPSP is normally ineffective in generating an impulse (cf. Figure 23D).

The simple exponential decay that is sometimes observed for the direct inhibitory curve (Lloyd, 1946; Laporte and Lloyd, 1952) is an unexpected finding in view of the double composition that has been demonstrated for inhibitory action. A probable explanation is that brief repetitive discharges of the intermediate neurones in the Ia inhibitory pathway would provide a continuing inhibitory action which would serve to retard the initial rapid decay of the inhibitory curve from its maximum. A single group Ia volley was found to evoke double or even triple discharges from some Ia intermediate neurones (Figure 59C,D,E). Such repetitive discharges are likely to be more common and more prolonged in Lloyd's unanaesthetized preparations.

4. Effects of Alterations of the IPSP

When the concentration of chloride or of other small anions such as nitrate or bromide in the motoneurone is sufficiently increased by injection from the microelectrode, the IPSP is converted from a hyperpolarizing to a depolarizing response (cf. Figures 40, 41). If the depolarization is sufficient, the IPSP will generate a spike discharge, the threshold level for this excitatory action being identical with that for the EPSP (Figure 41B,C,H). Not only has the increased anion concentration displaced the equilibrium potential for the IPSP to a smaller value than the resting potential, but an increase in the ionic fluxes occurring across the active inhibitory areas would also be expected; hence conditions should be more favourable for interaction between the inhibitory and excitatory responses. For example, in Figure 55D at an interval of

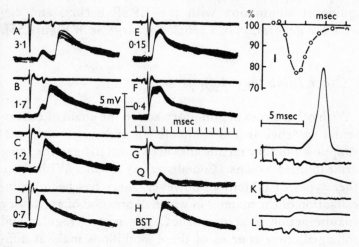

Figure 55

A–H. Series of records as in Figure 53 and for the same motoneurone, but after reversal of IPSP due to dosage with chloride. The volley intervals are marked on each record. *G* and *H* give control responses to quadriceps and to biceps-semitendinosus volleys alone. Voltage scale gives 5 mV for intracellular recording. *I.* Plot as in Figure 54B (open circles) for the heights of the EPSP's in subtracted records for series partly illustrated in Figure 55A–H. *J.–L.* Intracellular potentials produced by simultaneous IPSP and EPSP in a motoneurone heavily dosed with chloride. In *J*, summation of the two depolarizing responses generates a spike, whereas either alone fails in *K* and *L* respectively (Coombs, Eccles, and Fatt, 1955d).

0.7 msec., when the peaks of the IPSP and EPSP would be virtually synchronous, the combined response was very little larger than the control EPSP. If the potential added by the EPSP is calculated by subtraction as in Figure 54B, it is found that the apparent depression of the EPSP runs practically the same time course as in Figure 54B (open circles), but it is about 50 per cent larger (Figure 55I). The failure of the IPSP to add any appreciable depolarization to the summit of the EPSP (Figure 55D) indicates that the equilibrium potential for the IPSP is at a membrane potential very little more depolarized than the summit of the EPSP. When, by increasing the intracellular chloride concentration, the equilibrium potential for the IPSP is displaced further in the depolarizing direction, significant summation with the EPSP occurs, and can cause the generation of a reflex discharge as in Figure 55J.

5. Other Inhibitory Actions

With other types of inhibitory action the chain of experimental evidence is less complete. In every case the postsynaptic inhibitory membranes are shown to have the same permeabilities to ions (Coombs et al., 1955b). With these other types of inhibition, however, there has been no investigation of the manner in which depression of excitatory synaptic action is accomplished. The more irregular and prolonged time courses of these inhibitions make it difficult to carry out experiments of the type described in this chapter. Since the ionic mechanisms have been shown to be similar, however, it seems likely that any individual inhibitory synapse is effective in suppressing the reflex discharges from motoneurones by the same complex mechanism that has here been proposed for direct inhibition. If all inhibitory synapses are thus similarly effective on motoneurones, the differences between the various types of inhibitory action will arise on account of differences in the spatio-temporal pattern of the inhibitory bombardment.

6. Conclusions

It has been shown (Chapter III) that an inhibitory volley causes inhibitory subsynaptic areas of the motoneurone membrane to become highly permeable to K^+ and Cl^- ions. As a consequence of this brief increase of ionic permeability, which is at a high level for less than 2 msec., there is an outward current through these inhibitory areas, which hyperpolarizes the whole postsynaptic membrane, so producing the inhibitory postsynaptic potential. It is shown above that this increased ionic permeability has a double depressant action on the effectiveness with which excitatory synaptic action evokes the discharge of an impulse. It is further shown that the latent period and the time course of direct inhibitory action (the inhibitory curve) are accounted for satisfactorily. Finally, it is postulated that almost all the transmitter substance liberated from an inhibitory synapse is removed within two milliseconds from the region of its action on the postsynaptic membrane.

In conclusion, the schematic representation (Figure 56A) and the electrical circuit diagram (Figure 56B) give

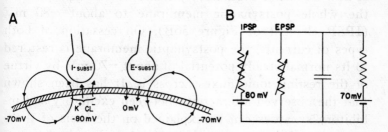

Figure 56

A. Schematic representation illustrating the manner of operation of an inhibitory and an excitatory synapse. One single line of current flow is drawn for each in order to illustrate the way in which the respective subsynaptic currents change the potential of the whole postsynaptic membrane in opposite directions. The voltages driving the inhibitory and excitatory currents are shown as −10 mV and +70 mV respectively (cf. Figure 52B). *B.* Formal electrical circuit diagram illustrating impedence elements and voltage sources in the motoneurone membrane. The right half of the diagram represents the condition of the general postsynaptic membrane, i.e., that part not covered by activated synapses, as has already been illustrated in Figure 9. The variable resistances represent the manner of operation of the inhibitory and excitatory subsynaptic areas. Direct inhibitory action causes the resistance of the inhibitory subsynaptic areas to fall as low as $7 \times 10^5 \Omega$ (cf. p. 120), while with monosynaptic excitatory action the corresponding resistance may be as low as $5 \times 10^5 \Omega$ (cf. Figure 22). In the absence of activation, these resistances would be so high that the currents through them have a negligible effect on the membrane, as is indicated by the open switch in Figure 22 (Coombs, *et al.,* 1955d).

in outline the essential features of operation of excitatory and inhibitory synapses and can serve as a basis for explanations of all observations on their action and interaction. An impulse reaching an excitatory synapse operates by liberation of a transmitter substance which causes a brief ionic current to flow inward across the subsynaptic membrane. By means of the lines of flow illustrated on the right of Figure 56A, this subsynaptic current tends to depolarize the whole postsynaptic membrane to about 0 mV (EPSP element of Figure 56B). If the current causes a depolarization by about 10 mV, an impulse is generated in the postsynaptic membrane of the initial segment (cf. Chapter II). Correspondingly, with the inhibitory synapse, an impulse liberates a transmitter which causes the subsynaptic membrane to generate a current (cf. line of flow on left of Figure 56A) that tends to hyperpolarize the whole postsynaptic membrane to about -80 mV (IPSP element of Figure 56B). On cessation of both types of currents, the postsynaptic membrane is restored to its normal steady potential of about -70 mV by virtue of the resting ionic fluxes across it. It has been shown that the observed interactions between excitatory and inhibitory synapses can be explained on the basis of these currents and the consequent potential changes in the postsynaptic membrane.

It has been proposed (Renshaw, 1946b; Howland, Lettvin, McCulloch, Pitts, and Wall, 1955) that an inhibitory volley exerts its effects by causing a depression of the size of the volley that is evoking the testing reflex, i.e., that inhibitory action is exerted at least in part presynaptically, and not postsynaptically. Experimentally it can be shown that an afferent volley set up by dorsal root stimulation causes a considerable diminution in the spike potential produced by a presynaptic volley in other afferent fibres (Brooks, Eccles, and Malcolm, 1948; Howland et al., 1955). This effect, however, is attributable to the dorsal root reflexes and the dorsal root potentials which are produced by large dorsal root volleys (Brooks et al., 1948). It has not been demonstrated with a volley of group Ia impulses, such as has been employed above. Furthermore, under natural conditions, as distinct from experimental, inhibition is produced by the repetitive asynchronous discharges of receptor organs, which provide a situation very unfavourable for causing such presynaptic blockage.

On the other hand, an inhibitory mechanism comprising the subsynaptic currents and the IPSP, as proposed above, is operated very effectively by repetitive asynchronous discharges of receptor organs. The relatively long duration of the IPSP gives opportunity for the spatial and temporal summation of the inhibitory effects produced on a motoneurone by such an inhibitory bombardment. It will be appreciated further that the effectiveness of this inhibitory mechanism will be greatly enhanced because naturally it will be exerted against a background depolarization produced by repetitive excitatory synaptic bombardment. For effective inhibition to occur, this depolarization has only to be maintained below the firing threshold. Under such conditions of depolarization, the inhibitory ionic currents will be greatly potentiated (cf. Figure 54A). With natural physiological conditions we have to envisage motoneurones as being subjected to a continuous bombardment by impulses impinging at both the excitatory and inhibitory synapses. The neurone discharges impulses only when the excitatory synaptic activity is momentarily so dominant that it causes the depolarization to attain the critical level (about 10 mV) for the initial segment.

B. CRUSTACEAN STRETCH RECEPTOR CELLS (KUFFLER AND EYZAGUIRRE, 1955)

The experimental situation with these cells differs from that of motoneurones because the interacting excitatory potential is produced not by synaptic action but by stretch deformation of the dendritic terminals. For example, in

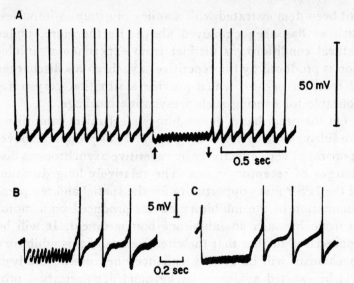

Figure 57

Intracellular recording from a crustacean stretch receptor cell of the slowly adapting type. *A*. The regular train of impulses (11 per sec.) set up by maintained stretch is interrupted by stimulation of the I axon, (cf. Figure 49A), between arrows, at 34 per sec. The small deflections are the repetitive IPSP's (cf. Figure 49B). *B, C*. Recording at higher amplification in order to illustrate the inhibitory action of the IPSP's, the frequencies of the inhibitory impulses being 34 per and 150 per sec. respectively. The initial discharges of the receptor cell at 4 per sec. are not shown, but this frequency is seen to be resumed promptly on cessation of the repetitive IPSP's (Kuffler and Eyzaguirre, 1955).

Figure 57A maintained stretch caused a regular train of afferent discharges, each arising when a slow depolarizing wave (the prepotential) reached a critical level. This discharge was immediately arrested by a train of inhibitory impulses (between the arrows) and returned on cessation of the inhibitory bombardment. It can be seen that the prepotential was suppressed during the inhibitory effect, which provides a sufficient explanation of the suppression of the afferent discharge. With the higher amplification of Figure 57 B,C, the repolarizing action of the inhibitory impulses can be seen either as discrete waves with low frequency (34 per sec.), or as a steady level of repolariza-

tion at high frequency (150 per sec.). No trace of a prepotential occurs during the inhibitory action, but it arises
immediately afterward.

Thus, afferent discharges normally are produced by a
"generator potential" in the stretched dendritic terminals,
which depolarizes the remainder of the dendrites and the
soma, so evoking the prepotentials which at a critical level
cause the discharge of impulses. The inhibitory action is
exerted primarily on the generator potential, i.e., inhibitory impulses control the afferent discharge in Figure 57,
not by suppression of conducted impulses, but by reducing
the generator potential. This inhibitory mechanism closely
resembles that of motoneurones, where inhibitory impulses also act by diminishing the excitatory depolarization.

C. GENERAL DISCUSSION

In both cases that we have considered, the inhibitory
impulses diminish the excitatory depolarization by making
the subsynaptic membrane highly conductive to certain
ions. With the crustacean receptor cell, this conductance
is so high that the membrane potential is virtually
"clamped" at the equilibrium potential for the inhibitory
ionic mechanism. Normally this equilibrium potential is
about 5 mV more depolarized than the completely relaxed
potential (cf. Figure 49B). The clamping of the membrane
potential at this slightly depolarized level (cf. Figure 57),
however, provides a very adequate inhibitory mechanism,
for a much larger depolarization of the dendrites (at least
20 mV) is required in order to generate an impulse (Eyzaguirre and Kuffler, 1955a,b). With motoneurones, inhibitory impulses do not produce such a high ionic conductance
of the postsynaptic membrane. Their effectiveness in coun-
teracting the excitatory depolarization arises because the
equilibrium potential of the inhibitory ionic mechanism is

about 10 mV more hyperpolarized than the resting potential. A larger battery compensates for a lower ionic conductance.

The important finding, however, is that inhibition is produced by essentially the same electrical mechanism in two such widely differing exemplars of inhibitory action. Furthermore, still more diverse tissues have now been shown to exhibit similar inhibitory mechanisms. Vagal inhibition of cardiac muscle is explained sufficiently by the repolarization of the surface membrane and the consequent suppression of the prepotentials that generate the propagated impulses, just as occurs in Figure 57 (Castillo and Katz, 1955c; Hutter and Trautwein, 1955). There is evidence that an increased K^+ ion conductance is produced by the vagal transmitter substance (Burgen and Terroux, 1953), but probably there is raised Cl^- ion permeability as well. Inhibitory impulses are also in part effective on crustacean muscle by virtue of an increased conductance for K^+ ions and also for anions, which presumably are Cl^- ions (Fatt and Katz, 1953). A large part of the inhibitory effect, however, appears to be due to a curare-like action of the inhibitory transmitter substance, which competes with the excitatory transmitter for the same receptor areas on the muscle membrane (Fatt and Katz, 1953). No trace of such a competitive mechanism has been detected with any other inhibitory action.

CHAPTER V

PATHWAYS AND SYNAPTIC TRANS-
MITTER SUBSTANCES IN THE
CENTRAL NERVOUS SYSTEM

Hitherto we have considered the behaviour of individual nerve cells, particularly as they are subjected to synaptic bombardment. We have not been concerned primarily with pathways traversed by impulses on their way to the nerve cells, in particular motoneurones, or with the transmitter mechanisms by which the activated presynaptic terminals evoke the excitatory or inhibitory postsynaptic responses of the nerve cells.

When considering the mode of operation of the nervous system and its relation to structure, however, there arises the important question: Do the branches of any one nerve cell exert an excitatory synaptic action on some neurones and an inhibitory synaptic action on others? A study of the inhibitory pathways to motoneurones is particularly germane to this question. The pathways for "direct" and "antidromic" inhibition have been investigated in detail and will be described before the data relating to various other pathways, both excitatory and inhibitory, are briefly presented. The monosynaptic excitatory pathway for collaterals from group Ia afferent fibres to motoneurones (cf. Chapter II) presents no features requiring special comment (cf. Cajal, 1909, Figures 113, 115; Schimert, 1939).

A. PATHWAYS IN THE CENTRAL NERVOUS SYSTEM

1. The Direct Inhibitory Pathway

In "direct inhibition," impulses from the annulo-spiral endings of a muscle inhibit the motoneurones of a muscle having antagonistic action (Lloyd, 1941b; 1946; Laporte and Lloyd, 1952; Bradley *et al.*, 1953). Until recently, values for the central conduction time of this pathway have been derived from measurements of the shortest interval at which an inhibitory volley can precede a monosynaptic excitatory volley and yet be effective in inhibiting the reflex discharge. Since such intervals approximated to zero, it was erroneously concluded that the latency of direct inhibitory action approximated to that of monosynaptic excitatory action, and hence that the inhibitory pathway was also monosynaptic, i.e., that the annulospiral afferents of muscle had inhibitory synaptic endings on motoneurones (Lloyd, 1946; Laporte and Lloyd, 1952; Brock *et al.*, 1952b; J. C. Eccles, 1953; Bradley *et al.*, 1953). Intracellular recording from motoneurones, however, has revealed that inhibitory synapses bring about inhibition by generating a hyperpolarizing response, the IPSP, of the motoneurone mêmbrane. The latent period for the onset of the direct IPSP gives an exact measurement of the central time for the inhibitory pathway, and shows that it is always much longer than the central time for monosynaptic excitatory action, as measured by the latency of the EPSP (cf. Figures 43A,C; 51I,J; 53H,I; 58A,B,D,E). Despite this longer latency, however, it can be shown that the IPSP is early enough to account for the observed direct inhibitory action (cf. Figure 52A).

Under some conditions, e.g., afferent impulses from quadriceps muscle inhibiting biceps-semitendinosus motoneurones (Figure 58A,B), the inhibitory path must travel longitudinally in the spinal cord even for more than 1 cm. However, after any longitudinal intramedullary conduction time in the inhibitory pathway has been measured and allowed for (cf. the reverse allowance for Figure 58D,E), the central latency for the IPSP generated by direct inhibitory action is about 0.8 msec. longer than for the monosynaptic EPSP (Eccles, Fatt, and Landgren, 1956). A possible explanation of this longer latency would be that it occurs between the arrival of the inhibitory impulses at the presynaptic terminals and the generation of the IPSP. Extracellular recording in the immediate

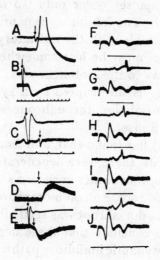

Figure 58

A, B. Intracellular recording from a biceps-semitendinosus motoneurone at upper S1 level, showing EPSP and IPSP responses to afferent volleys from biceps-semitendinosus and quadriceps nerves respectively. The EPSP in *A* rises quickly to a spike. Latent periods (0.55 msec. and 1.45 msec., respectively) are measured from the arrows on the accompanying spike potentials of the afferent volleys as recorded by a contact electrode on L6 dorsal root. Time, msec. All records of Figure 58 are made by superposition of about 40 faint traces. *C.* Extracellular recording at higher amplification and faster speed just outside motoneurone of *A, B,* downward deflexion being negative both for dorsal root and extracellular records. The latent period of the spike attributable to inhibitory presynaptic terminals (1.1 msec.) is measured between the two arrows. Time, msec. *D, E.* Intracellular recording of EPSP and IPSP responses evoked by the same afferent volleys in a presumed knee flexor motoneurone at upper L6 level (probably a gracilis motoneurone). Extracellular recording showed that the initial, less steeply sloped deflexion in *E* is due to the potential field of the focal synaptic potential generated by adjacent quadriceps motoneurones, the IPSP beginning at the arrow. Time, as for *B.* *F–J.* Upper record of each pair shows extracellularly recorded potentials from the intermediate nucleus at lower L6 level, while lower record shows potentials simultaneously evoked on the dorsolateral aspect of cord at upper L7 level. Stimulus setting up quadriceps afferent volley was progressively increased from *F* to *J,* being maximal for group Ia fibres at *I.* Note extracellularly recorded synaptic potential (EPSP) in intermediate nucleus and single spike superimposed thereon in *G–J.* Upward deflexions signal increasing negativity for both sets of records. Time, msec. (Eccles, Fatt, and Landgren, 1956).

neighbourhood of the inhibited motoneurones, however, reveals that spike potentials (Figure 58C) generated by the inhibitory impulses occur only 0.3 msec. before the onset of the IPSP. The inhibitory synaptic delay thus has a duration comparable with the excitatory synaptic delay, and the 0.8 msec. must be lost somewhere on the direct inhibitory pathway to the motoneurones; hence, it is likely that this pathway is interrupted by a synaptic relay, for the delay in transmission through one synapse occupies approximately 0.8 msec.

Sprague (1956) has found that, 3 to 5 days after sectioning cat dorsal roots, there were degenerating fibres ending synaptically on motoneurones even two segments removed from the sectioned root, e.g., on motoneurones in S_1 and L_7 segments when L_5 dorsal root was sectioned. It is not justified, however, to conclude that these degenerating fibres belong to a monosynaptic inhibitory pathway, for it has now been shown that a sufficient explanation is provided by primary afferent fibres entering the spinal cord through L_5 dorsal root and establishing monosynaptic excitatory connections with motoneurones in the L_7 and S_1 segments, quadriceps afferent fibres so ending on soleus motoneurones and gracilis afferent fibres on semitendinosus motoneurones (Eccles, Eccles, and Lundberg, unpublished observations). Anatomical evidence, therefore, has not established that there are any monosynaptic connections in the direct inhibitory pathway.

Exploration with a microelectrode has established that the primary afferent impulses in the fibres from annulo-spiral endings synaptically excite special neurones of the intermediate nucleus of Cajal, and that the properties of this synaptic relay conform with known properties of the direct inhibitory pathway (Eccles, Fatt, and Landgren, 1956). For example, some intermediate neurones discharge impulses with a latency as brief as 0.8 msec. (Figure 59C) and have a very low threshold for discharge, as well as a high safety factor and an ability to respond to high frequencies of synaptic stimulation—even over 600 a sec.

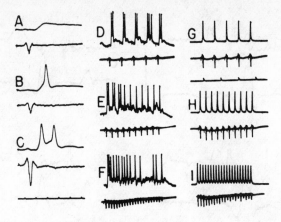

Figure 59

A, B, C. Intracellularly recorded responses evoked from a neurone of the intermediate nucleus by a quadriceps afferent volley. The afferent volley was progressively increased in size from *A* to *C*. The lower records give the action potential recorded by a contact electrode on the L6 dorsal root for each strength of stimulus. Spikes are upward in intracellular records and downward with dorsal root records. Time, msec. *D, E, F.* Intracellular and dorsal root recording, as above, but to repetitive quadriceps afferent volleys, the respective frequencies being 145, 330, and 650 per second. *G, H, I.* Same experiment as above, but the intracellular recording was from a group Ia quadriceps afferent fibre in the intermediate nucleus. Repetitive stimulation as in *D–F*, and at same frequencies. Time scale in 10 msec. between *G* and *H* obtains for *D* to *I* (Eccles, Fatt, and Landgren, 1956).

(Figure 59F). Furthermore, the observed selectivity of the direct inhibitory function (cf. Lloyd, 1946; Laporte and Lloyd, 1952) would be preserved despite propagation across this synaptic relay. The primary group Ia afferent impulses from any one muscle excite a specific group of intermediate neurones (group Ia intermediate neurones) that are not excited by such impulses from muscles other than synergists, or by any impulses from Golgi tendon organs (cf. Figure 60). As shown in Figure 61, however, many intermediate neurones that are thus selectively excited by group Ia impulses are also excited by group III muscle impulses (B,C,D) and by cutaneous impulses (E,F). This functioning of group Ia intermediate neurones

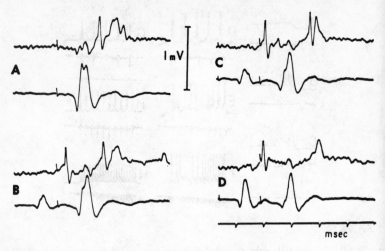

Figure 60

In *A*, a quadriceps afferent volley set up by a stimulus just maximal for groups Ia and b (see double spike in the lower trace recorded by a surface electrode on the L6 dorsal root) evoked responses of at least three neurones which were recorded extracellularly by a microelectrode in the intermediate nucleus (upper record), the first giving a sharp diphasic spike. In *B–D* this constant testing stimulus was preceded at a fixed interval of 1.5 msec. by a conditioning stimulus of progressively increasing intensity. With *B*, the conditioning volley was large enough to evoke a discharge from the intermediate neurone giving the sharp diphasic spike; nevertheless, this neurone discharged again in response to the testing volley, as also occurred in *C*. In *D*, a further increase in the conditioning volley prevented the testing volley from evoking a discharge, though it was maximum for group Ib impulses and was effective for the later discharges, i.e., the diphasic spike was activated only by the group Ia volley, which was fractionated in *B* and *C*. Upward deflexions signal negativity in all records. Voltage scale gives 1 mV for microelectrode records (Eccles, Fatt, and Landgren, 1956).

as a common path for other afferent modalities does not conflict with any experimental evidence relating to the specificity of the direct inhibitory path.

It may be assumed that the group Ia fibres send collaterals into the intermediate nucleus as described by Cajal (1909, Figures 113, 115) and by Schimert (1939). Intracellular or extracellular recording from a single intermediate neurone reveals that the collaterals of several group Ia fibres converge onto it. As a consequence, graded

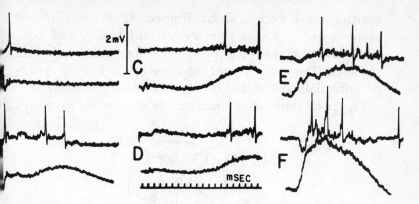

Figure 61

Upper trace gives extracellular recording (as in Figure 60) from an intermediate neurone excited by impulses in group Ia fibres of quadriceps nerve. Lower trace gives recording by a surface electrode from the L6 dorsal root. In *A*, the quadriceps volley was maximum for group Ia. In *B*, it was maximum for groups I to III. *C* and *D* were evoked by gastrocnemius-soleus and plantaris afferent volleys respectively, both including groups I to III: *E* and *F* were evoked by superficial peroneal and sural volleys respectively, which also included all the medullated fibres. Time scale applies to all records. Voltage scale applies to records from intermediate nucleus (Eccles, Fatt, and Landgren, 1956).

EPSP's are set up just as in motoneurones, and one or more impulses are generated if the EPSP is sufficiently large (Figure 59 B,C). The more intense the EPSP, the briefer is the delay involved in generating an impulse.

Systematic exploration of the potential fields in the spinal cord has shown that impulses appear in the inhibitory presynaptic terminals (Figure 58C) almost immediately after the intermediate neurones discharge impulses, but their axonal pathway has not been revealed by this procedure. Further evidence relating to the axonal pathway is provided by the brief positive wave that is produced on the dorsolateral regions of the spinal cord as current flows from the somas of the intermediate neurones into the activated presynaptic inhibitory terminals in the motoneuronal nucleus (Eccles, Fatt, and Landgren, 1956). As shown in the lower records of Figure 58F–J, this brief positive wave occurs about 1 msec. after the triphasic spike potential of the primary afferent volley, and both potentials increase together with increasing stimulus strength. The upper records of Figure 58F–J show synaptic potentials and spikes of an intermediate neurone.

Figure 62 shows diagrammatically the central pathways

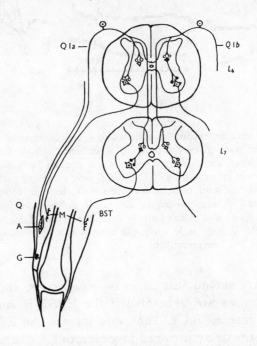

Figure 62

Diagram showing the postulated pathways with L6 and L7 segments for impulses entering the spinal cord along group Ia and Ib afferent fibres from the quadriceps muscle. The synaptic connexions of the Q Ia fibres are shown in the left halves and those of the Q Ib fibres in the right halves of the two transverse sections. Excitatory nerve cells and synaptic knobs are drawn as open structures and inhibitory cells and knobs are filled in. Q = quadriceps muscle; BST = biceps and semitendinosus muscles; M = motor nerve endings; A = annulo-spiral ending in a muscle spindle; G = Golgi tendon organ. (modified from Eccles, Fatt, Landgren, and Winsbury, 1954).

that have been revealed by these experiments. The large afferent fibres from the annulo-spiral endings of quadriceps muscle (A) are seen to end monosynaptically around motoneurones belonging to their synergic group of muscles and to send collaterals down to intermediate neurones in L7 segment (cf. Cajal, 1909, Figures 113, 115), which complete the direct inhibitory pathway by sending their axons to the motoneurones of antagonistic muscles (biceps-semitendinosus). It is presumed that these latter axons are medullated, because negative spike potentials have not been detected along their course (Eccles, Fatt, and Landgren, 1956). By the bouton-degeneration method, Szentágothai (1951) has found that some short propriospinal fibres from the intermediate nucleus form synaptic articulations with motoneurones, which conforms with the pathway here postulated.

The anatomical pathway and the physiological events occurring along it can now be summarized in a diagram (Figure 63), which shows the way in which converging

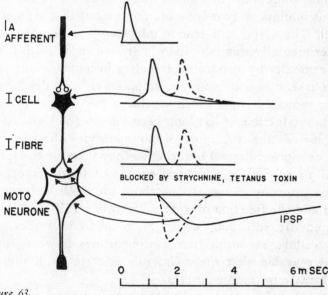

Figure 63

Schematic drawing of the anatomical and physiological features of the direct inhibitory pathway. It shows the events in the primary afferent fibre, in its excitatory synaptic connections with an intermediate neurone (I cell) and finally in the inhibitory synaptic connection of this neurone with a motoneurone, where the inhibitory subsynaptic current is shown by a broken line and the IPSP by a continuous line (cf. Figure 36A).

afferent impulses evoke, by means of excitatory synaptic action, the discharge of one or two impulses from an intermediate cell. These impulses in turn exert an inhibitory synaptic action on the motoneurone, so generating the IPSP. This diagram gives a precise account of the time relationships of the various events. Thus, the intermediate neurone discharges an impulse within 1 msec. of the time of entry of the afferent volley into the spinal cord, and the inhibitory potential begins about 0.3 msec. after the arrival of this impulse at the motoneurone.

2. The Antidromic Inhibitory Pathway

In 1941 Renshaw gave the first description of "antidromic inhibition," in which a volley of impulses in motor axons inhibits all types of motoneurones at that segmental level. The term "antidromic inhibition" is used because experimentally this inhibition is evoked most readily and conveniently by antidromic impulses in motor axons, but, of course, it is also evoked by impulses reflexly discharged from motoneurones, which would be the normal manner of its production. It has long been known (cf. Cajal, 1909, pp. 363-67) that the axons of motoneurones often give off one or more collateral branches as they traverse the spinal cord to emerge in a ventral root, and there have been many interesting suggestions about the mode of termination and the function of such collaterals (cf. Jung, 1953a). Systematic recording along microelectrode tracks and intracellular recording from motoneurones, however, have now revealed that the collaterals operate an inhibitory pathway onto motoneurones.

Impulses in motor axons set up a prolonged repetitive discharge of a unique group of interneurones in the ventromedial region of the ventral horn, as was first described by Renshaw (1946a). It can be shown that the activation of these interneurones (now designated "Renshaw cells") is not caused by impulses propagating over the somas and dendrites of motoneurones; it is therefore postulated that their activation takes place via the collaterals of motor axons (Eccles, Fatt, and Koketsu, 1954). As demonstrated by the extracellular records from a single Renshaw cell (Figure 64B), collaterals from many motor axons of different functions converge onto it and excite the discharge of impulses, the initial frequency being usually over 1000 a second (Figure 64A). Intracellular recording shows that the impulses arise from a background depolarization of the Renshaw cell (Figure 64F,G), which can be seen to have a duration of at least 50 msec. when it is not complicated by superimposed impulses (Figure 64I).

In conformity with the principle first enunciated by Dale (1935) that the same chemical transmitter is released from all the synaptic terminals of a neurone, pharmacological investigation has indicated that acetylcholine mediates the excitation of Renshaw cells by impulses in the collaterals of motor axons, just as it mediates the excitation of muscle fibres at the peripheral terminals of the same axons. For example, the responses of Renshaw cells to synaptic stimulation are depressed by drugs such as dihydro-β-erythroidine, which block cholinergic transmission (Figures 64C and 65H), and are greatly prolonged by anticholinesterases such as eserine and TEPP (Figures 64D; 65D), while the intra-arterial injection of acetylcholine and of nicotine directly excites Renshaw cells (Figure 65B,C). As would be expected, the excitatory action of acetylcholine, but not nicotine, is increased by anticholinesterases (Figure 65E,F,G), while dihydro-β-erythroidine decreases the excitatory action of both substances (Figure 65I,J). Some drugs, however, exhibit anomalous action on this presumed cholinergic junction. For example, D-tubocurarine always fails to depress transmission, while prostigmine has usually only a very slight anticholinesterase action, and acetylcholine may have no detectable excitatory action. There is evidence that prostigmine is blocked by the blood-brain barrier (Eccles, Eccles, and Fatt, 1956), which may also account for the ineffectiveness of the other

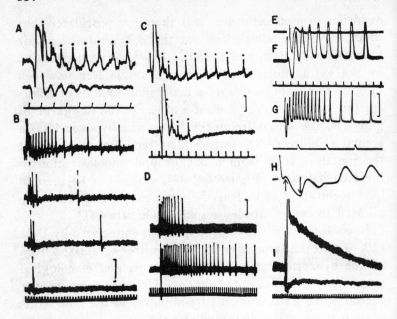

Figure 64

A. Upper record shows the rhythmic response set up in an interneurone by an antidromic volley in the biceps-semitendinosus motor axons. The eight brief spikes (indicated by dots) generated by this interneurone are seen superimposed on complex waves formed by superimposed spikes of other interneurones. The large initial diphasic wave is generated by the antidromic volley as it approaches and then invades the biceps-semitendinosus motoneurones. The lower tracing is recorded by a surface lead on the dorsolateral aspect of the cord. Time, msec. *B.* Upper record as in *A,* but with slower sweep speed, in order to show full duration of interneuronal response. Other records, from above downward, responses of same interneurone elicited by antidromic volleys in the motor axons to gastrocnemius, flexor longus digitorum, and the deep peroneal group of muscles, respectively. Time, msec. Potential scale, 0.5 mV. *C.* As in *A,* but interneuronal spikes (indicated by dots) elicited by an antidromic volley in the L7 ventral root. Upper record before and lower record after intravenous injection of 0.1 mg/Kg of dihydro-β-erythroidine hydrobromide. The rhythmic response continued far beyond the ten spikes of the upper series, whereas after injection it ceased after the four spikes. Time, msec. Potential scale, 0.5 mV. *D.* As in *C,* but at much slower sweep speed, to show in upper record full duration of repetitive interneuronal spikes evoked by an antidromic volley in the L7 ventral root. Lower record after injection of 0.1 mg/Kg of the anticholinesterase, NU.2126, the spike series continuing even beyond 0.45 second. Time, 10 msec. Potential scale, 0.5 mV. *F* to *H* are the responses evoked in another Renshaw cell by a maximum volley in L7 ventral root and recorded intracellularly, upward deflection indicating positivity of microelectrode rela-

quaternary substances, D-tubocurarine and acetylcholine.
Intracellular recording from motoneurones in the lumbar region of cat spinal cord has revealed that a volley of

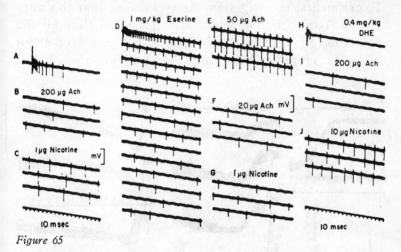

Figure 65

Responses of another Renshaw cell. There was no spontaneous discharge. *A* is response to a single antidromic volley in L7 ventral root, while *B* and *C* each show three successive sweeps at the height of the responses evoked by intra-arterial injection of 200 μg of acetylcholine and 1 μg of nicotine, respectively. Several minutes after the intravenous injection of 1.0 mg eserine/kg, the response *A* was changed to *D*, while *E*, *F* and *G* show, respectively, three successive records at the heights of the responses evoked by the intra-arterial injections of 50 μg acetylcholine, 20 μg acetylcholine and 1 μg nicotine. Records *H*, *I*, and *J* were obtained during the maximum of the depression produced by the intravenous injection of 0.4 mg dihydro-β-erythroidine hydrobromide/kg, H being evoked by the antidromic volley and I and J by the intra-arterial injections of 200 μg acetylcholine and 10 μg nicotine, respectively (Eccles, Eccles, and Fatt, 1956).

tive to the indifferent electrode, i.e., it is the reverse of other figures in which the Renshaw cell discharges have been recorded extracellularly. Three different sweep speeds are used as shown by the msec. time scales for *F* and *H*, *G* speed being one third of that for *F*. Smaller responses in *H* are due to progressive failure of cell. Latent period is measured between the two arrows, the initial response evoked by the antidromic volley being extracellularly recorded and so being inverted. Note that the second of the four Renshaw cell responses is so early that it is greatly reduced in size. Potential scale gives 5 mV. *I* shows potentials recorded inside (cf. *F–H*) and just outside another Renshaw cell at much slower sweep speed (see time scale in msec.). Amplification 5 times that for *F–H*. (Eccles, Fatt, and Koketsu, 1954).

impulses in motor axons generates a hyperpolarization of
the motoneuronal membrane that has all the features of an
inhibitory postsynaptic potential (Figures 38, 39B, 44B).
Experimental investigation has established that this antidromic IPSP of motoneurones is produced through the
mediation of Renshaw cells. The latent period of about
1.5 msec. (Figure 66A,C) and the prolonged time course

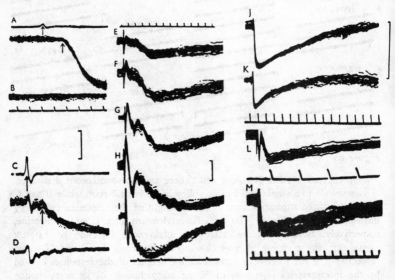

Figure 66

Intracellular recording (with superposition of about 40 faint traces) of
the IPSP's produced by an antidromic volley in L7 ventral root in all but
records *B* and *D*, which were obtained extracellularly for the motoneurones
generating potentials *A* and *C*, respectively. The IPSP is given by the difference between the two potentials and so commences at the second arrow.
Above the intracellular potentials of *A* and *C* are also the surface potentials
which signal (at first arrow) the time of entry of the antidromic volley into
the spinal cord, i.e., the latent period for the IPSP is the interval between
the two arrows in *A* and *C*. Time in msec. Series *E–H* shows IPSP's produced
by progressively larger antidromic volleys. With *H* and *I* the volley is maximum, *I* being at a much slower sweep as indicated by 10 msec. time below.
J, K. Effect of injecting 0.1 mg dihydro-β-erythroidine hydrobromide/kg body
weight in diminishing and shortening duration of the IPSP from J to K. Time
scale in 10 msec. *L, M.* Effect of injection of 0.3 mg eserine sulphate/kg body
weight in lengthening duration of the IPSP from L to M. Note that sweep is
almost four times slower for M, as shown by respective 10 msec. time scales.
(Eccles, Fatt, and Koketsu, 1954).

of the IPSP (Figure 66I,J) are in precise accord with this explanation. It is particularly convincing that the antidromic IPSP often exhibits a high frequency ripple (about 1000 a sec.) corresponding to the initial high frequency of the Renshaw cell discharge (cf. Figure 66H). Furthermore, depression and shortening of the Renshaw cell discharge by dihydro-β-erythroidine and its prolongation by anticholinesterases are accompanied by corresponding changes in the antidromic IPSP as shown by Figure 66J,K and Figure 66L,M, respectively. The reflex inhibitory effect that is produced by the antidromic IPSP has been fully investigated by Renshaw (1941).

The proposed anatomical pathway is shown in the enlarged inset of Figure 67B. Motor axon collaterals converge onto and make excitatory synaptic contacts with Renshaw cells whose axons in turn converge onto and make inhibitory synaptic contacts with motoneurones at the same segmental level. Systematic mapping of the electric potential fields in the spinal cord reveals that Renshaw cells are concentrated in the ventromedial region of the ventral horn of the spinal cord and send their axons dorsolaterally to the motoneurones, as shown in Figure 67B. The repetitive spike potentials which an antidromic volley generates in the population of Renshaw cells are initially so well synchronized that they fuse and give a rhythmic potential wave at about 1000 per sec., which is a prominent feature in records from the surface of the spinal cord (cf. lower record of Figure 64A). When recorded in the dorsolateral regions of the spinal cord (upper five records of Figure 67A), this wave has a polarity which is the inverse of the polarity in the ventromedial zone (lower three records of Figure 67A), where it arises from the repetitive discharges of Renshaw cells. This orientation of the potential field is attributable to the dorsolateral path of the axons from the Renshaw cells, as shown in Figure 67B.

The physiological events in the antidromic inhibitory pathway are shown diagrammatically in Figure 68. The single volley in the motor-axon collaterals (A) liberates

acetylcholine from its synaptic terminals with time course
(B), and so generates, after a latency of about 0.6 msec.,

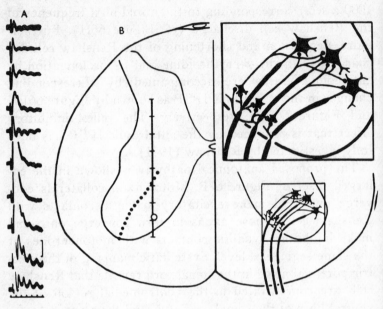

Figure 67

A. Potentials recorded from the L7 segment of the spinal cord in response to a maximum antidromic volley in the L7 ventral root. Each record
is formed by the superposition of about 40 faint traces. The uppermost
record is by a surface lead from the dorsolateral surface. The remaining
records are obtained at the depths indicated by short transverse lines along
the track shown by the continuous line running dorsoventrally on the left
side of Figure 67B. Time is in msec. Potential scale gives 0.5 mV for all
but the uppermost record, where it gives 0.05 mV. Upward deflections signal
negativity of recording electrode relative to the indifferent lead. *B.* Drawing of a transverse section of the spinal cord. In the left half, the open circle
indicates the maximum focus of Renshaw cell activity as detected by systematic exploration. Also shown is the electrode track along which records
of *A* were recorded. The dotted line separates the ventromedial zone of
Renshaw cell negativity from the dorsolateral zone of Renshaw cell positivity. On the right half is shown in schematic form the proposed nervous
pathways (see details in inset above) consisting of motor-axon collaterals,
Renshaw cells, and motoneurones. The Renshaw cells are located in the
region from which most recordings from individual cells were obtained and
their axons course therefrom to the motoneurones in the direction that
accounts for the phase reversal of the rhythmic wave generated by their
discharges (see text) (Eccles, Fatt, and Koketsu, 1954).

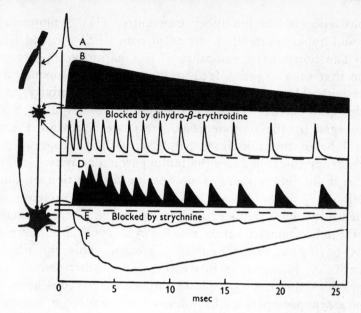

Figure 68

Diagram summarizing the postulated sequence of events from an impulse in a motor axon to the inhibition of a motoneurone. All events are plotted on the time scale shown below and the corresponding histological structures (cf. Figure 67B) are shown diagrammatically to the left (note indicator arrows). The six plotted time courses are for the following events: *A*, the electrical response of impulse in motor-axon collateral; *B*, the effective concentration of the acetylcholine which it liberates at a synaptic terminal; *C*, the electrical response evoked in a Renshaw cell by the cumulative effect of acetylcholine at many synapses, showing impulses superimposed on a background depolarization (cf. Figure 64F); *D*, the effective concentration of inhibitory transmitter substance which these impulses liberate at a synaptic terminal of the Renshaw cell, showing summation at the high initial frequency; *E*, the IPSP generated in the motoneurone by the Renshaw cell discharge and the inhibitory transmitter shown in *D* and *C*, respectively; *F*, the aggregate IPSP evoked in a motoneurone that is bombarded repetitively by many Renshaw cells, which become progressively more asynchronous, so smoothing the latter part of the ripple shown in E. The structural diagram to the left shows converging synapses both on the Renshaw cell and on the motoneurone (cf. Figure 67B) (Eccles, Fatt, and Koketsu, 1954).

a repetitive discharge of a Renshaw cell (C), which de-clines progressively in frequency. After a further latency of about 0.6 msec. this discharge generates through the mediation of the inhibitory transmitter (D), a motoneuronal hyperpolarization, the antidromic IPSP (E and F).

The functional significance of this pathway appears to be that of a negative feed-back control of motoneuronal activity. The more intense this motoneuronal activity, i.e., the greater the frequency and number of impulses discharged by the motoneurone, the more activation there will be of this inhibitory pathway, with the consequent tendency to damp down the motoneuronal activity. Unlike direct inhibition there is no specific distribution of this inhibitory action to one functional kind of motoneurone, hence it cannot fulfill a coordinative action. There is a general indiscriminate action which can be considered merely as having an anticonvulsant function. This inhibitory pathway, however, is interesting for another reason. It provides the first example in the central nervous system of a synapse operated by a known transmitter substance, in this case, acetylcholine.

3. Pathways for Afferent Fibres of Golgi Tendon Organs (Group Ib Fibres)

Laporte and Lloyd (1952) have shown that group Ib impulses have actions on motoneurones which are reciprocally antagonist to those exerted by group Ia impulses, and that they also have other inhibitory actions not falling into this category. The latent periods of these actions led to the postulate that both the excitatory and inhibitory pathways for group Ib impulses are disynaptic, having just one interneurone. This evidence needs reassessment. The disynaptic character of the group Ib inhibitory pathway was postulated because it was believed to have a latency that was one synaptic delay longer than the direct inhibitory pathway, which is itself now known to be disynaptic.

When the whole transverse section of the spinal cord is explored systematically by a series of parallel insertions of a microelectrode, it is found by extracellular recording that the group Ib primary afferent impulses produce excitatory postsynaptic potentials only in the region of the ipselateral intermediate nucleus (Eccles, Fatt, Landgren and Winsbury, 1954). As recorded extracellularly, these group Ib EPSP's resemble the group Ia EPSP's of this nucleus, differing only in the longer latent period. When the discharges of individual intermediate neurones can be recognized, the latent period is found to be about 0.3 msec. longer than for the discharges from group Ia intermediate neurones (cf. Figure 60A). In part, this longer delay is attributable to the longer conduction time in the peripheral pathway (up to 0.2 msec.; cf. Bradley and Eccles, 1953), but it seems that a longer synaptic delay also must be postulated.

Finally, the latency of the IPSP produced by the relayed Ib afferent impulses can be measured by intracellular recording from motoneurones. With the reciprocal type of group Ib action, the IPSP will be superimposed on a monosynaptic EPSP, which makes a direct reading of the IPSP latency an inaccurate procedure. The origin of the IPSP from the background EPSP can be detected precisely if Cl^- ions are injected into the neurone or if the motoneuronal membrane potential is altered by current applied through one barrel of a double microelectrode. As shown in Figure 69 A,B, the IPSP is greatly changed by the Cl^- injection, while the EPSP is unaltered. It is also much more affected than the EPSP by alterations of the membrane potential Figure 69C-G. The latency so measured for the IPSP generated by group Ib impulses is 1.5 msec. Latencies of 1.5 msec. to 2 msec. also are observed when the IPSP is not superimposed on a preceding EPSP. Thus, our observations are in good agreement with those of Laporte and Lloyd (1952) in showing that group Ib inhibition has a latency that is approximately 0.5 msec. longer than group Ia inhibition. Most of this difference has been shown to occur in the respective latencies of the intermediate cell discharges which are set up by the primary afferent volleys (cf. Figure 60A). When measured from the time of the

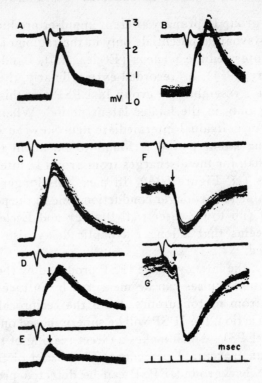

Figure 69

Lower records show intracellular responses (superposition of about 40 faint traces) of a plantaris motoneurone to a maximum group I volley in plantaris afferent fibres, as shown in upper records. After record *A,* approximately 50 p. mole of Cl^- ions were run into the cell electrophoretically, the subsequent response, B, being not changed significantly until after the arrow, where evidently an IPSP response was converted from a hyperpolarizing to a depolarizing type. *C–G* shows that a similar separation of the EPSP from the IPSP component is achieved by varying the membrane potential as in Figures 20, 37, and 38. The initial monosynaptic EPSP response was only reversed to a hyperpolarizing response with the depolarization of *F,* while the later IPSP component was reversed between *D* and *E,* the respective reversal potentials being about +10 mV and −20 mV. All indicator arrows are drawn at 1.5 msec. after the arrival of the plantaris volley at the spinal cord.

corresponding intermediate cell discharges, the respective latent periods of the IPSP's show at most a difference of 0.2 msec., which is far too brief for an additional synapse. It may, therefore, be concluded that even as the group Ia inhibitory pathway is disynaptic, so is the group Ib inhibitory pathway (cf. Figure 62 at L6 level). The intermediate group Ib neurones must exert their inhibitory action directly on the motoneurones, just as has been found to occur for the group Ia intermediate neurones.

Likewise, in agreement with Laporte and Lloyd (1952), group Ib impulses can be shown to exert excitatory actions on motoneurones, i.e., to generate EPSP's, by a disynaptic pathway involving intermediate neurones (cf. Figure 62 at L7 level). Presumably these neurones are different from those responsible for the inhibitory action.

4. Segmental Reflex Pathways for Other Primary Afferent Fibres

The experimental evidence relating to cutaneous afferent fibres is very incomplete. Most of the synaptic relays occur in the dorsal horn (Coombs, Curtis, and Landgren, 1956). Both large and small cutaneous fibres have been found to excite the same intermediate neurones that relay group Ia impulses (Figure 61E,F). Also they excite repetitive discharges from other intermediate neurones that seem to be specialized for the cutaneous pathway (Figure 70A,B,C). Group III muscle afferent impulses also have synaptic relays in the dorsal horn and excite some intermediate neurones of inhibitory function that relay group Ia impulses (Figure 61C,D) as well as neurones that relay cutaneous impulses.

5. Afferent Projection Pathways

In those pathways where the synaptic relays have been investigated thoroughly, the synaptic mechanism with one exception has resembled that described above for segmental reflex pathways. This new feature is provided by the very powerful excitatory action exerted by single pre-

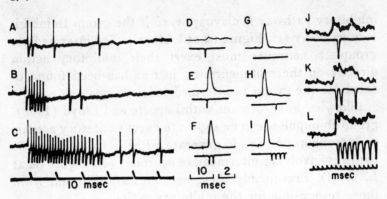

Figure 70

A–C. Responses of an intermediate neurone recorded as in Figure 61 and evoked by an afferent volley in sural nerve, which was evoked by stimuli which were, respectively, 2, 8, and 40 times threshold. *D, E, F.* Upper traces are samples of the afferent volley from quadriceps nerve as recorded monophasically from a dorsal root filament. Lower traces are slower intracellular records from a fibre of the dorsal spinocerebellar tract showing spikes evoked by the corresponding afferent volley. Note different time scales. *G, H, I.* Similar series of records, but from another fibre of the dorsal spinocerebellar tract, which was not activated by a maximum group I volley from quadriceps nerve (*G*), but was activated by group II (*H*) and group III volleys (*I*). *J, K, L.* The lower trace again shows spikes intracellularly recorded from a fibre of the dorsal spinocerebellar tract, but the upper trace is a monophasic record from the tract in the mid-thoracic region. The afferent volley was from superficial peroneal nerve, the stimulus strength being increased from *J* to *L.* (Laporte, Lundberg, and Oscarsson, 1956).

synaptic impulses. The three synaptic relays that have been investigated most thoroughly will serve to illustrate this feature.

By stimulating various afferent nerves and recording the responses of single fibres of the dorsal spinocerebellar tract, Laporte, Lundberg, and Oscarsson (1956) have shown that some tract fibres are activated specifically by impulses from muscle spindles, both group Ia and group II. A very small group Ia volley in Figure 70D caused the discharge of a single impulse, which also was observed with a maximum group Ia volley (E). Strengthening the stimulus sufficiently to add the group II volley caused the addition of a second impulse (F). Other tract fibres are not activated by group I impulses (Figure 70G), but discharge singly in response to a group II volley (H) and repetitively when a group III volley also is added (I). Still other tract fibres are specifically activated by cutaneous impulses. The impulses of lowest threshold evoke the discharge of one or a few impulses (Figure 70J,K), while cutaneous volleys set up by stronger stimuli give a repetitive discharge with a frequency as high as 1000 per sec. (Figure 70L). These last two types of fibres can be regarded as components of one main group, because each often receives subsidiary activation by the afferent fibres of the other.

The group Ia or II volleys evoke discharges of single impulses with synaptic delays of less than 1 msec. In contrast, the repetitive discharges evoked by group III impulses from muscle and by cutaneous volleys resemble the discharges which cutaneous volleys evoke from interneurones (Figure 70B,C). This discrimination of tract fibres into two classes was not appreciated by previous investigators (Grundfest and Campbell, 1942; Lloyd and McIntyre, 1950), but otherwise there is no inconsistency with their results. For example, Lloyd and McIntyre found that a dorsal root volley evoked a prolonged repetitive discharge, and concluded, largely on the basis of threshold levels, that it was produced by the group I afferent fibres of muscle. Presumably even their weakest stimulation of the dorsal roots was exciting cutaneous afferents as well as muscle afferents. There is general agreement that the cells of origin of the dorsal spinocerebellar tract, i.e., the neurones of Clarke's column, are excited to discharge impulses by a very few group Ia afferent impulses. The histological correlate of this powerful synpatic excitatory action of single impulses is revealed in the remarkable "giant synapses," in which synaptic contact apparently is made for several hundred microns along dendrites as well as in the giant terminal end bulbs, so giving areas of contact of many hundred square microns (Szentágothai and Albert, 1955). Such synaptic contacts are very many times larger than any made by the branched ending of a single presynaptic fibre on a motoneurone. Degeneration experiments show that several different afferent fibres form giant synapses with a single cell. This correlates with the physiological evidence that the same tract fibre can be activated by afferent volleys from different muscle nerves and that thereby the synaptic relay has potentially a coordinative function (Grundfest and Campbell, 1942; Laporte, Lundberg, and Oscarsson, 1956). In addition, Szentágothai and Albert (1955) describe smaller synaptic endings on the cells of Clarke's column, some apparently originating in interneurones in the dorsal horn and others as collaterals from spinocerebellar tract fibres. Possibly some of these contribute to the repetitive responses evoked by cutaneous volleys and by group III afferent volleys from muscle (cf. Grundfest and Campbell, 1942). Presumably also some of these accessory endings are concerned with the inhibitory synaptic action which has been demonstrated to occur with both types of neurones of Clarke's column (Laporte, Lundberg, and Oscarsson, 1956).

As with Clarke's column, single impulses in dorsal column fibres have a powerful excitatory action on the neurones of the cuneate and gracile nuclei, a single impulse probably being adequate to evoke a discharge with a synaptic delay as brief as 0.6 msec. (Therman, 1941; Amassian and DeVito, 1956). Correspondingly, single afferent fibres make very extensive synaptic contacts, though apparently not with giant synapses as in Clarke's column (Glees and Soler, 1951). In addition, there is convergence of afferent fibres onto the same cell (cf. Glees and Soler, 1951), their conjoint action shortening the latent period and causing a repetitive response at high frequency. Probably, as suggested by Amassian, repetitive discharge also results from the action of impulses in the axon collaterals that are distributed to adjacent neurones (cf. Cajal. 1909, p. 902). There is no evidence of interneuronal activity.

There has been an intensive investigation of the synaptic relay in the dorsal nucleus of the lateral geniculate body between optic nerve fibres and the cells of origin of the optic radiation (G. H. Bishop and O'Leary, 1940; 1942; P. O. Bishop, 1953; P. O. Bishop, Jeremy, and McLeod, 1953; P. O. Bishop and McLeod, 1954; Tasaki, Polley, and Orrego, 1954). Again, as with the other afferent projection pathways, single afferent impulses have a powerful excitatory action. The discharge of impulses in the optic radiation is observed even with the smallest volleys in the optic nerve. When special measures are adopted to suppress this discharge, however, a focal synaptic potential is recorded which runs a time course that is virtually identical with that given by motoneurones, the latent period being 0.3 msec. to 0.4 msec., and the total duration about 4 msec. (P. O. Bishop, 1953; P. O. Bishop and McLeod, 1954). Thus, in many features the synaptic relay in the lateral geniculate body resembles that of the monosynaptic reflex pathway. The principal differences arise because of the much more powerful excitatory actions of single afferent impulses, and also, in the repetitive discharge that is often evoked from the lateral geniculate body, probably because of the activity of both axon collaterals and interneurones (P. O. Bishop, Jeremy, and McLeod, 1953).

In summary, it can be stated that these afferent projection pathways all show a powerful synaptic excitatory action of single impulses and a limited amount of convergence, so that there is not a 1 to 1 relationship of impulses across the synaptic junction. It appears that the synaptic relays in the afferent pathway thus subserve some integrative function, particularly as there are superimposed synaptic actions by axon collaterals and by interneurones. It is of interest that there is no convincing example of an inhibitory action at the synaptic relays in the gracile and cuneate nuclei and in the lateral geniculate body. With repetitive stimulation there is depression of the secondary discharges, but probably this is merely an example of the depressions that have already been described with repetitive presynaptic volleys.

6. Descending Pathways in the Spinal Cord
(Lloyd, 1944)

The synaptic relays of these pathways have not yet been studied in sufficient detail to provide valuable information on the synaptic mechanisms. In general, the only statements that can be made relate to the cells which are synaptically excited by volleys in the descending tracts. For example, Lloyd (1941c) has shown that, in the cat, volleys descending the pyramidal tract excite discharges from cells at the base of the dorsal horn and in the intermediate nucleus, which in turn act upon the motoneurones either directly or by further interneurones, though usually this has been observed only after several volleys of a repetitive series. On the other hand, Granit (1955, Figure 126) finds that the application of single stimuli to cat motor cortex may evoke twitch-like responses from leg muscles, though it is not clear if this is due to monosynaptic or to polysynaptic action of the pyramidal tract volley. There is a close parallelism between these physiological results and anatomical investigation by the bouton-degeneration method. In the cat, synaptic endings of the pyramidal tract are profuse on the cells at the base of the dorsal horn and there are very few on motoneurones (Hoff, 1932b; 1935; Szentágothai-Schimert, 1941; Szentágothai, 1951). In the monkey, a considerable proportion of the synaptic endings of pyramidal tract fibres are on motoneurones (Hoff and Hoff, 1934), and correspondingly it has been shown that pyramidal tract volleys activate motoneurones monosynaptically (Bernhard, Bohm, and Peterson, 1953). Monosynaptic discharges usually are evoked only after the facilitatory action of several pyramidal volleys at 10 to 20 a sec. Single pyramidal volleys, however, facilitate monosynaptic segmental reflexes by direct synaptic action on motoneurones. Both anatomical and physiological evidence indicate that most of the pyramidal tract endings are on interneurones.

In the cat, almost all synaptic endings of the ventrolateral tracts also occur on interneurones, which in turn relay to motoneurones. The physiological investigations of Lloyd (1941a) are in agreement with the results of Schimert (1938); Szentágothai-Schimert (1941; 1951) using the bouton-degeneration method. Similarly the long propriospinal tracts end in synaptic relationship with interneurones in the intermediate and ventral horns (Lloyd, 1942; Szentágothai, 1951).

An explanation of the facilitatory influence of repetitive stimulation of the motor cortex and other higher centres is provided by the associated discharges from small motoneurones to the muscle spindles, which are thus in turn stimulated to fire the excitatory group Ia impulses back to the large motoneurones (Granit and Kaada, 1952; Granit, 1955, cf. Figure 126). Evidence of such an action was illustrated by Lloyd (1941c, Figure 12). Presumably also the flower-spray endings on muscle spindles would be discharging group II impulses (Hunt, 1954), which appear to act primarily on the interneurones of the spinal cord (Coombs, Curtis, and Landgren, 1956). Therefore, in order to assess the excitatory influence which is exerted on interneurones and motoneurones by volleys in the descending pathways, it is necessary to eliminate the muscle spindle afferents by dorsal root section, a procedure which so far has been adopted only rarely.

It might be considered that the fine discriminative movements characteristic of pyramidal tract activity would have been produced more effectively if the pyramidal fibres had exclusively made direct synaptic articulations with large motoneurones. Such an arrangement, however, presumably would have restricted pyramidal action to a purely excitatory role, for it may be assumed that activation of the special inhibitory cells is necessary for inhibition. Presumably, therefore, some of the interneurones on the pyramidal pathway to motoneurones are inhibitory cells. A similar assumption may be made for other descending pathways, e.g., from the cerebellum, the red nucleus, and the reticular formation. More generally, it can be stated that, by establishing synaptic connections with interneurones rather than with motoneurones, the pyramidal tract and the other descending tracts are able to operate through the coordinative mechanisms at the segmental levels of the spinal cord (Lloyd, 1944; Austin, 1952).

B. SUBSTANCES MEDIATING SYNAPTIC TRANSMISSION BETWEEN NERVE CELLS

Until recently there were two tenable explanations of the transmission mechanism for synaptic excitatory and inhibitory action (cf. Bremer, 1951; Fessard and Posternak, 1950): (1) that it was due to the flow of electric currents generated by presynaptic excitatory impulses; (2) that it was due to the postsynaptic action of transmitter substances that were liberated by presynaptic impulses. Because of the following experimental evidence the first of these alternatives has now become untenable (cf. the comprehensive review by Fatt, 1954).

(a) Intracellular recording has shown that presynaptic impulses cause no detectable potential change in the postsynaptic membrane (Brock *et al.*, 1952a), even with the synapse between giant axons of *Loligo* (Figure 34; Bullock and Hagiwara, 1956). The observed potential changes, the EPSP or IPSP, begin after the summit of the presynaptic spike potential, i.e., during the rising phase of the presynaptic spike potential there is no detectable potential change across the postsynaptic membrane. Hence, only a negligible fraction of the presynaptic current can penetrate the postsynaptic membrane.

(b) When the potential of the postsynaptic membrane has been diminished by extrinsic current, the EPSP has changed correspondingly, the EPSP even being reversed when the membrane potential is reversed (Figures 20, 21, 23A). The electrical transmission hypothesis cannot offer an explanation of these observations, whereas they are readily explained by the chemical transmitter hypothesis (Coombs *et al.*, 1955c and Chapter II).

(c) The monosynaptic EPSP of a motoneurone is generated by a depolarizing current that is in excess of 1×10^{-7}A (cf. discussion in relation to Figure 22), which is about 50 times the total current at the node of a medullated fibre (Huxley and Stampfli, 1949; Tasaki, 1953; 1955). Since the group Ia fibres from a muscle are less numerous than the motoneurones of that muscle, the convergence of many group Ia fibres onto one motoneurone can occur only because there is an equivalent branching of the group Ia presynaptic fibres. One motoneurone would be subjected to the excitatory currents flowing back from the synaptic knobs to nodes further upstream on the presynaptic fibres. The aggregate of these currents would not be greater than the total current generated by one node on the parent group Ia afferent fibre, which would be about 2×10^{-9}A (Huxley and Stampfli, 1949; Tasaki, 1953; 1955). It seems that, even if the presynaptic fibre could very effectively inject its currents across the postsynaptic membrane, it would fail by a factor of at least fifty to produce the required current. It was proposed that the injected current could be amplified by a local response mechanism (Eccles, 1946b), but the effect of reversal of the membrane potential in reversing the EPSP makes this suggestion untenable (Figure 20). With the end-plate potential of amphibian muscle, the presynaptic impulse fails by a factor of thousands to provide the depolarizing current required to generate the observed end-plate potential (cf. Fatt and Katz, 1951).

(d) On the basis of an electrical transmission hypothesis (cf. Brooks and Eccles, 1947a), it has been impossible to offer an explanation for the hyperpolarization (the IPSP) which inhibitory impulses induce in the postsynaptic membrane (cf. Brock *et al.*, 1952a).

(e) Variation of the postsynaptic membrane potential by extrinsic current caused large changes, even reversal, of the IPSP (cf. Figures 37, 38, 39). These changes have been readily explicable in terms of a special ionic permeability that the inhibitory transmitter substance induces in the subsynaptic membrane. No explanation could be possible in terms of any electrical transmitter hypothesis.

(f) Similarly the effects produced in the IPSP by changes in the ionic composition of the motoneurone (Figures 37, 38, 40, 41, 47) are readily explicable in terms of ionic permeability changes of the subsynaptic membrane, but are inexplicable in terms of any electrical transmitter hypothesis.

Already a considerable theoretical structure has been erected on the basis of chemical transmitter mechanisms across synapses. The experimental evidence classified above gives assurance in finally rejecting the possibility of electrical transmission. It is proposed now to consider the evidence relating to the synaptic transmitter substances.

1. Acetylcholine as the Transmitter Substance

a. At synapses of sympathetic ganglia

It should not be necessary to do more than summarize, under the five headings below, the experimental evidence which establishes the cholinergic nature of synaptic transmission in sympathetic ganglia and which has been reviewed often (Dale, 1935; 1937; Brown, 1937; Eccles, 1936b; Bronk, 1939; Feldberg, 1945; 1950a; 1950b; Fessard and Posternak, 1950; Fatt, 1954; Minz, 1955). In addition, there is now good experimental evidence that acetylcholine is also the synaptic transmitter in parasympathetic ganglia (Emmelin and Muren, 1950; Perry and Talesnik, 1953).

(i) Preganglionic fibres contain a store of acetylcholine that is manufactured by their choline-acetylase system, which also effectively replenishes the store when it is depleted by activity.

(ii) Preganglionic impulses cause the liberation of acetylcholine from this store (Emmelin and MacIntosh, 1956).

It can be calculated that under optimal conditions a single preganglionic volley liberates up to 10^{-15}g around one ganglion cell (Eccles, 1953).

(iii) Very low concentrations of acetylcholine are effective in depolarizing ganglion cells and evoking the discharge of impulses from them. The threshold concentration is as low as 5×10^{-8} when there is adequate anticholinesterase (Emmelin and MacIntosh, 1956).

(iv) Specific cholinesterase is concentrated on the preganglionic fibres (Koelle, 1954). Investigation of the effects produced by its inactivation by anticholinesterases reveals that it hydrolyses the liberated acetylcholine, so limiting the accumulation around ganglion cells and possibly also making choline available for the further synthesis of acetylcholine by the preganglionic terminals (Perry, 1953).

(v) Drugs such as D-tubocurarine and its analogues very effectively depress the excitatory action both of preganglionic impulses and of acetylcholine on ganglion cells. Since the liberation of acetylcholine by preganglionic impulses is unaffected, the synaptic blockage is sufficiently explained by the depression of the excitatory action of the liberated acetylcholine.

The convincing character of this evidence is apt to give assurance that there are no outstanding problems in ganglionic transmission. Suggestions of unresolved problems, however, are indicated by the electrical responses of deeply curarized ganglia. The initial excitatory postsynaptic potential is then negligible, but it is followed first by a large hyperpolarizing potential (the P wave) and second by a depolarization (the LN wave) having several seconds' duration (Laporte and Lorente de Nó, 1950; R. M. Eccles, 1952b; 1956).

As suggested by Laporte and Lorente de Nó, the P wave is probably due to the inhibitory synaptic action of specific preganglionic fibres. Its pharmacological properties indicate that this presumed inhibitory transmission is not mediated by acetylcholine. On the other hand, the LN wave is depressed very effectively by all anticholine-

sterases, though not by D-tubocurarine and its analogues
(R. M. Eccles, 1952b; 1956). It is suggested that the LN
wave is produced by a new type of cholinergic transmission, acetylcholine depolarizing the ganglion cells by acting on special receptor areas having a cholinesterase
configuration. If these areas are a little removed from the
synaptic terminals, the LN wave would be expected to
have the long latency that is observed. The possibility
must be envisaged, therefore, that a single transmitter
substance may have two completely different receptor
surfaces on the same subsynaptic membrane. Despite this
difference, the ultimate effect on the postsynaptic membrane is the same, e.g., depolarization in the example
illustrated.

b. *Motor-axon collaterals to Renshaw cells*

The evidence that this synaptic transmission is mediated
by acetylcholine has already been presented. It is the first
example of a specifically defined cholinergic synaptic
mechanism in the central nervous system, and is also of
interest as an example of Dale's principle, which postulates the identity of chemical transmission from the diverse
branches of a neurone. It seems likely that other central
cholinergic synaptic mechanisms will have similar pharmacological properties. If that is so, the excitatory action of
nicotine (Figure 65C) and the depressant action of
dihydro-β-erythroidine (Figures 64C, 65H,I,J) should be
of particular significance in the experimental attempt to
locate these synapses.

There is general agreement that, when administered by
intravenous or intra-arterial injection, nicotine depresses
monosynaptic reflexes such as tendon jerks, and that acetylcholine has a similar action when given intra-arterially
or even intravenously, if the cholinesterase is inactivated
(Schweitzer and Wright, 1937a,b; 1938; Bulbring and Burn,
1941; van Harreveld and Feigen, 1948; Taugner and Culp,
1953; Curtis, Eccles, and Eccles, 1955). The depression
appears in 1 sec. to 3 sec. after the beginning of an intra-

arterial injection of acetylcholine and has disappeared by 10 sec. (Figure 71A,B). With nicotine there is a similar latency, but longer duration (Figure 71A,C). Since these drugs evoked discharges from Renshaw cells, which in turn

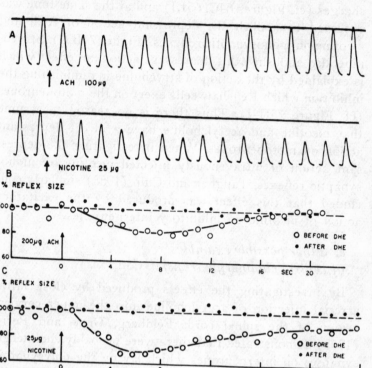

Figure 71

A. Monosynaptic reflex spikes were evoked by L7 dorsal root volleys at a frequency of 1 per sec. and recorded monophasically in the L7 ventral root. The individual spikes had a duration of about 1 msec., but the brief gaps between each represent about 1 sec. In the upper series, the arrow signals close intra-arterial injection of 100 μg of acetylcholine, which results in a depression of the reflexes for about 10 sec. In the lower series, 25 μg of nicotine sulphate produced a more profound and lasting depression, recovery occupying about 60 seconds. The horizontal lines were formed by the other beam, which was adjusted at the mean summit heights for a long series of reflex spikes immediately before the injection. *B, C.* The open circles plot measurements for series such as those of A, while the filled circles show the complete abolition of depression after the intravenous injection of 0.8 mg of dihydro-β-erythroidine hydrobromide (DHE)/kg body weight (Curtis, Eccles, and Eccles, 1955).

inhibited motoneurones, it was possible that the observed depression was brought about in this way. A crucial test was provided by the action of dihydro-β-erythroidine, which very effectively diminished the Renshaw cell discharges (cf. Figures 64C, 65I,J) and at the same time was observed to abolish the depressant action of ACh and nicotine on monosynaptic reflexes (Figure 71B,C). Strychnine also abolished this depressant action, an effect which is explained by the action of strychnine in diminishing the inhibition which Renshaw cells exert on the motoneurones (cf. Figure 73G–J). Thus there is no reason to assume that nicotine and acetylcholine have a direct depressant action on motoneurones. When investigating the depressant action of intravenously injected nicotine on monosynaptic reflexes, Taugner and Culp (1953) similarly concluded that this effect was produced by the excitatory action of nicotine on inhibitory interneurones.

c. Other possible examples of central cholinergic transmission

By investigating the effects produced by close intra-arterial injection of acetylcholine into the upper cervical region of the spinal cord, Feldberg, Gray, and Perry (1953) demonstrated that there were probably cholinergic synapses on interneurones which lay on the polysynaptic reflex pathways from dorsal to ventral root. It is generally agreed that dorsal root fibres themselves are not cholinergic in their central synaptic action (Eccles, 1948; Bremer, 1953a; Feldberg, 1954), a conclusion that conforms with the very low acetylcholine and choline-acetylase content of dorsal root fibres (MacIntosh, 1941; Feldberg, 1945; Feldberg and Vogt, 1948).

The systematic examination of the choline-acetylase activity of diverse parts of the central nervous system has shown that some regions have high activity (Feldberg and Vogt, 1948) and that the distribution corresponds with that determined for acetylcholine (MacIntosh, 1941; Feldberg, 1945). There is, furthermore, reasonable correlation with the distribution of specific cholinesterase (Burgen and Chipman, 1951; Koelle, 1954), hence it has been postulated that cholinergic synaptic activity is exerted by the neurones of the regions rich in the three components of the acetylcholine system (Feldberg and Vogt, 1948; Burgen and Chipman, 1951; Koelle, 1954). For example, the neurones of the cuneate and gracile nuclei and of the lateral geniculate body would exert a cholinergic synaptic action on the neurones next in series. Little weight can be given to this postulate unless it is supported by a thorough pharmacological and neurophysiological investigation of the synaptic transmission.

It seems likely that there are also cholinergic synapses in the cerebral cortex, for MacIntosh and Oborin (1953) find that considerable quantities of acetylcholine (up to 6×10^{-9}g cm^{-2}min.$^{-1}$) are liberated into the fluid exuding from active cerebral cortex, while none can be detected with the deeply anaesthetised cortex. It is suggested that the acetylcholine is produced by afferent fibres to the cortex, which have yet to be identified. Fibres from the lateral geniculate body may provide one source (cf. Feldberg and Vogt, 1948), and Marrazzi (1953) has produced evidence indicating that acetylcholine may be the excitatory transmitter substance for transcallosal fibres to the cortex.

2. Other Excitatory Transmitting Substances

In the investigation of synaptic transmission to motoneurones many pharmacological agents have been tested against diverse types of reflexes. In particular there have been frequent attempts to discriminate between the actions of drugs on monosynaptic and polysynaptic reflexes.

There has been general agreement that large doses of Myanesin (Mephenesin, Tolserol) selectively depress polysynaptic reflexes, monosynaptic reflexes being much less affected (Henneman, Kaplan, and Unna, 1949; Kaada,

1950; Taverner, 1952; Wright, 1954). It is possible that the observed decreases of monosynaptic reflxes are secondary to a depression of the background interneuronal discharges, and that Myanesin has no direct action on monosynaptic reflexes. If the action of Myanesin is restricted to synapses in interneuronal pathways, it may be taken to indicate that their synaptic transmitter differs from that operative in the monosynaptic pathway. Alternatively, Wright (1954) has suggested that Myanesin has a similar depressant action on both types of synapse, the greater depression of the polysynaptic reflexes arising because of the arrangement of the depressed synapses in serial order.

The action of strychnine is complementary to that of Myanesin, polysynaptic reflexes being greatly increased, while the monosynaptic reflexes are much less increased or even decreased (Hoffman, 1922; Bremer, 1944; Kaada, 1950; Naess, 1950; Bernhard, Taverner, and Widen, 1951; Scherrer, 1952; Brooks and Fuortes, 1952). It has been suggested (Bradley, Easton, and Eccles, 1953) that the monosynaptic reflexes are changed only in so far as there is a change in the background barrage of impulses on motoneurones and that the large increase in polysynaptic reflexes is attributable to the depression of inhibitory control at synaptic relays on this pathway. It is thus possible to explain the effects of strychnine on spinal reflexes by the only specific action which it is known to have on central synapses, namely, depression of the effectiveness with which activated inhibitory synapses generate the inhibitory postsynaptic potential (cf. Figure 73). The similar effects of brucein and thebaine on reflexes also are explained by the depression of inhibitory synaptic action. Such convulsants as picrotoxin and metrazol are not effective in this way. A possible explanation of their convulsant activity and also of that of strychnine and brucein has been suggested by Hellauer and Umrath (1948) and by Umrath (1953a), who find that all these convulsants very effectively inhibit an enzyme which destroys an "excitatory substance" extracted from dorsal roots.

A wide variety of possible transmitting substances or their analogues, when given by close intra-arterial injection, has no significant effect on monosynaptic reflexes. For example, adrenaline, noradrenaline, 5-hydroxytryptamine, histamine, caffeine, mecholyl, carbachol and succinylcholine were ineffective even in doses as large as 200 μg (Curtis, Eccles, and Eccles, 1955). When drugs were so administered intra-arterially, it was assumed that changes beginning many seconds (10 sec. to 30 sec.) after the injection, such as the increased reflexes often observed with adrenaline (cf. Skoglund, 1952), were due, not to a direct action on the synaptic mechanism, but to an action secondary to some other action of the injected substance, e.g., an alteration in the blood supply to the spinal cord arising because of a vasomotor response. Another complication with intra-arterial injection arises because of the action of some drugs (acetylcholine, nicotine, histamine, succinylcholine, and, possibly, 5-hydroxy-tryptamine) in evoking discharges from receptor organs (Brown and Gray, 1948; Armstrong, Dry, Keele, and Markham, 1953; Granit, Skoglund, and Thesleff, 1953) which would modify reflexly the monosynaptic reflexes. This complication can be eliminated by crushing the dorsal roots at the appropriate segmental levels.

When these various indirect actions of drugs are rejected, it appears that there is no good evidence for a direct and specific pharmacological action on the monosynaptic reflex pathway. It is certainly a surprising situation that a chemical transmitting mechanism has no pharmacology. Moreover, with the possible exception of ATP, it has not yet been possible to extract from the central nervous system a substance which has an excitatory action on central neurones when it is injected into the circulation. It is possible that the blood-brain diffusional barrier (Patek, 1944; Tschirgi, 1952; Woollam and Millen, 1954; Rodriguez, 1955) may account for these negative results from injection into the blood stream. Direct injection into the extracellular spaces should be attempted.

Following a suggestion by Dale (1935) that the substance causing antidromic vasodilation at the peripheral terminals of sensory fibres would probably be the transmitter substance at their central terminals, there has been intensive study of this vasodilator action. There is general agreement that extracts of dorsal roots have a vasodilator action on the standard test object, the ear of the rabbit, but it appears that the effective substances differ according to the method of extraction. For example, Holton and Holton (1954) have produced very strong evidence, both biochemical and pharmacological, that the effective substance in their extracts of dorsal roots and also of the caudate nucleus is largely adenosinetriphosphate, ATP. On the other hand, Hellauer and Umrath (1948), Umrath (1953a), and Hellauer (1953) have been extracting a substance that is certainly not ATP, but which may contain substance P, a polypeptide, as one active principle. There is no experimental evidence that this extracted substance has any central excitatory action, though it is called "Erregungssubstanz der sensiblen Nerven" because of the above suggestion of Dale (1935). On the other hand, ATP has been shown to stimulate the discharge of impulses from the spinal cord when it is given by intra-arterial injection in a rather large dose (Buchthal, Engbaek, Sten-Knudsen, and Thomasen, 1947), and other evidence of central stimulating or depressing actions was also given by Holton and Holton (1954). Much more precise evidence of synaptic excitatory action would be necessary, however, before ATP can be considered as a likely central transmitting substance.

The distribution of substance P throughout the central nervous system suggests that it could be a transmitting substance for the primary afferent nerve fibres, as first suggested by Lembeck (1953). Thus it occurs in relatively high concentration in the dorsal roots, the dorsal columns, and the grey matter of the spinal cord, and it is particularly concentrated in the gracile and cuneate nuclei (Pernow, 1953; Kapera and Lazarini, 1953; Amin, Crawford, and Gaddum, 1954), a distribution which would indicate a concentration in the synaptic terminals of the primary afferent fibres. Substance P also occurs in high concentration in various other parts of the central nervous system, e.g., the nuclei of the mesencephalon and hypothalamus and the corpus striatum, whereas it is in very low concentration in other parts, e.g., ventral roots, optic nerves, the cerebellum, and most of the cerebral cortex. This variability of distribution also has been observed for acetylcholine and choline-acetylase, and it suggests that substance P may likewise be a central synaptic transmitter substance. Unfortunately, this suggestion is subject to the grave objection that hitherto substance P has not been observed to exert any action on the central nervous system (Feldberg, 1954). Possibly, when given intravascularly, it is blocked by the blood-brain barrier. It should, therefore, be tested by direct injection into the neighbourhood of cells that are excited by primary afferent impulses.

Umrath (1953b) has provided evidence that the substance P extracted from gut may not be the same as that extracted from the nervous system (cf. Lembeck, 1953). The latter may be related to the "Erregungssubstanz," and Florey (1954) also suggests that the substance E which he extracts from the central nervous system may be identical with substance P. Evidently much further investigation is needed in order to clear up the confused position that at present exists in respect to the various extracts from dorsal roots and the central nervous system.

Adrenaline, noradrenaline, and 5-hydroxy-tryptamine are three related substances that occur in many parts of the central nervous system in parallel concentration, noradrenaline being almost always the most abundant and adrenaline the least (Vogt, 1954; Amin *et al.*, 1954). For example, highest concentrations occur in the hypothalamus, the area postrema, and the mid-brain, while there are very low concentrations in much of the cerebral hemisphere, the cerebellum, the dorsal and ventral roots. Since high concentrations are observed in parts of the nervous system devoid of nerve cells, the area postrema and gliomas, Vogt (1954) is led to suggest that these substances probably have some role other than synaptic transmission. She further points out that the experimental evidence on central actions of these substances fails to allow for secondary effects due to vascular changes. Their central concentration in areas associated functionally with the sympathetic system may indicate some other function (Vogt, 1954; Amin *et al.*, 1954). On the other hand, Marrazzi (1953) and Marrazzi and Hart (1955) find that, when given by intra-arterial injection, adrenaline, noradrenaline, and 5-hydroxy-tryptamine all have a depressant action on the negative phase of the diphasic potential wave which is generated in the cerebral cortex by a transcallosal volley, and suggest that all three substances have a synaptic inhibitory function. The long latent period of this depressant action (about 30 sec.), however, suggests that some secondary action is involved, e.g., anoxia due to vasoconstriction, though Marrazzi and Hart give evidence against this interpretation. Similarly, the striking effects produced by intra-arterially injected adrenaline on monosynaptic and polysynaptic reflexes had such a long latent period that they are likely to be secondary to vascular effects (Bernhard and Skoglund, 1953).

It may be concluded that central synaptic transmitter substances have not yet been satisfactorily shown to be present in the various extracts from the nervous system. Moreover, with the exception of acetylcholine, none of the known substances in extracts (adrenaline, noradrenaline, 5-hydroxy-tryptamine, substance P, histamine (cf. Parrot, 1954)) has yet been shown to function as a central synaptic transmitter. Such a demonstration would require more refined investigation, as, for example, local injection of the test substance into the immediate environment of the nerve cell whose responses are being recorded by a microelectrode. Feldberg and Sherwood (1954) have attempted to evade the obstruction by the blood-brain barrier by injecting substances intraventricularly, but the application of the drug is very widely dispersed and it is difficult to evaluate the significance of the complex behavioural responses that are produced in this way.

3. Inhibitory Transmitter Substances

When strychnine is injected intravenously in a subconvulsive dose, e.g., 0.1 mg/Kg, it greatly diminishes the amount of inhibition produced by a directly inhibiting volley, but has no significant effect on the testing monosynaptic reflex (Bradley *et al.*, 1953). For example, the inhibitory curve of Figure 72A was changed to that of

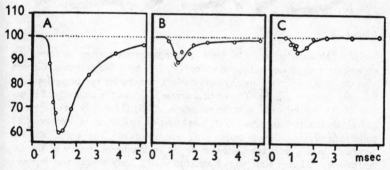

Figure 72

A. Inhibitory curve plotted as in Figure 50. B. Inhibitory curve after intravenous injection of 0.09 mg strychnine/kg body weight. C. Inhibitory curve after a further injection of 0.08 mg strychnine/kg body weight (Bradley, Easton, and Eccles, 1953).

Figure 72B. The further change to the curve of Figure 72C was produced by a second injection. Strychnine similarly diminishes the IPSP produced by any type of inhibitory action on motoneurones, but has no effect on the EPSP. For example, the direct IPSP of Figure 73A was converted to that of Figure 73D, while the monosynaptic EPSP was unaltered (Figure 73 B–E). Likewise the antidromic IPSP of Figure 73 G–J was diminished by approxi-

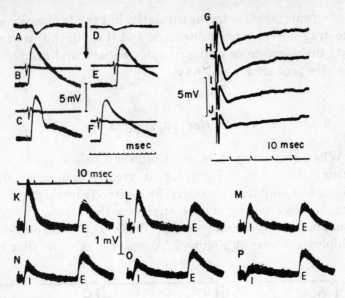

Figure 73

A–F. Intracellular records from a biceps-semitendinosus motoneurone evoked by a quadriceps afferent volley (*A, D*), by a biceps-semitendinosus afferent volley (*B, E*), and by both volleys, the quadriceps being later by 0.6-msec. interval (*C, F*). The vertical arrow indicates the intravenous injection of 0.1 mg/kg of strychnine salicylate, *A, B, C* being before injection and *D, E, F* after injection. *G–J.* The effect of strychnine in depressing an antidromic IPSP. Single traces only are recorded. The potentials are generated in a quadriceps motoneurone by an antidromic volley in the L6 ventral root. 0.1 mg. strychnine hydrochloride/kg body weight was injected intravenously between G and H. H–J were recorded at 10, 20, and 30 sec. after the injection. Maximum depression was attained at *J*. Time is in 10 msec. Potential scale, 5 mV. *K–P.* Intracellular recording of biceps-semitendinosus motoneurone whose Cl⁻ ion concentration was greatly increased by diffusion out of the microelectrode. In all records the initial response (I) is an IPSP of depolarizing type evoked by a quadriceps Ia volley and the later response (E), a monosynaptic EPSP. 0.1 mg/kg of strychnine salicylate was intravenously injected after *K* and the records *L–O* were recorded at successive intervals of 10 sec. thereafter. Record *P* was recorded after full development of the inhibitory depression produced by a second injection of 0.1 mg/kg of strychnine salicylate (Coombs, Eccles, and Fatt, 1955d; Eccles, Fatt, and Koketsu, 1954).

mately the same amount. Usually an injection of 0.1 mg/Kg reduces IPSP's of all types to about one-third. Strychnine also diminishes the IPSP when it is converted to a depolarizing response by increase in the intracellular chloride concentration. For example, Figure 73 K–O shows the progressive diminution of the IPSP, while the EPSP remains unaffected, and P gives the effect of a further injection. Conceivably strychnine could depress the inhibitory action by blocking the excitatory synaptic action on the inhibitory neurones which are interpolated in the inhibitory pathway. This possibility has been excluded by the observation that there is no diminution in the electrical responses which are produced on the surface of the spinal cord by activity of these inhibitory neurones, both those on the direct and those on the antidromic inhibitory pathway.

The highly specific and rapid action of strychnine in such relatively low doses suggests that it is acting in a manner resembling D-tubocurarine at the neuromuscular junction, i.e., that it acts competitively with the inhibitory transmitter for the receptor patches of the inhibitory subsynaptic membrane. In other words, we may regard strychnine as the "curare" of the inhibitory synapse—at least for five types of inhibitory action on motoneurones. Brucein has a similar, but less potent, action, as also has thebaine (Fatt, 1954). On the other hand, such convulsant drugs as picrotoxin and metrazol have no appreciable depressant action on the inhibitory synaptic mechanism in the spinal cord.

In general, the clinical effects produced by the actions of tetanus toxin and of strychnine are very similar, and on this account Sherrington (1906, pp. 109-13) suggested that these two substances acted similarly on the central nervous system. Experimental investigation (Brooks, Curtis, and Eccles, 1955) has confirmed this suggestion. For example, Figure 74 shows that an injection of tetanus toxin into the sciatic nerve produced after some hours a progressive diminution of inhibitory action on motoneurones on the ipsilateral side and later on the contralateral side. The long latency is attributable to the slow diffusion of tetanus toxin up the sciatic nerve. When it was injected

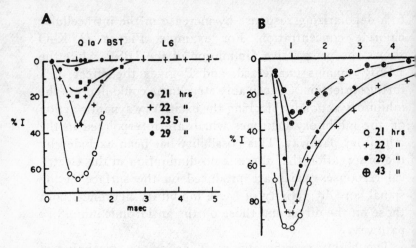

Figure 74

Curves as in Figures 50 and 72 showing time courses of direct inhibition of monosynaptic reflex from biceps-semitendinosus motoneurones of the spinal cord under Nembutal anaesthesia. The symbols denote the inhibitory effects observed at the times indicated after the injection of 7 mg of tetanus toxin (Wellcome XB 1322. T.166) in 0.05 ml normal saline under the sheath of the left sciatic nerve at the mid-thigh level. A and B were obtained on the left and right sides, respectively. Each plotted percentage is the mean of ten to twenty observations. (Brooks, Curtis, and Eccles, 1955).

into the spinal cord, the latency was reduced to a few minutes.

Just as was observed with strychnine, such doses of tetanus toxin have insignificant actions both on monosynaptic reflexes, and on the responses of the inhibitory neurones which lie on the inhibitory pathways. Hence, it can be assumed that tetanus toxin acts in a similar way in depressing the process whereby impulses in the synaptic terminals of these inhibitory neurones generate an IPSP of motoneurones. Possibly tetanus toxin might act in the manner postulated for strychnine and combine sterically with the special receptors of the subsynaptic inhibitory areas. In view of the general similarity of tetanus and botulinum toxin (van Heyningen, 1950), a possible alternative is that it acts like botulinum toxin at the neuromuscular junction (Brooks, 1956) and "seals" the inhibitory presynaptic terminals so that little or no transmitter substance is liberated therefrom.

Tetanus toxin also resembles strychnine in that it greatly increases polysynaptic reflexes. Possibly this effect may be similarly explained by the assumed depressant action on inhibitory synapses upstream along the polysynaptic pathway.

The similarities of the actions both of strychnine and of tetanus toxin on the various types of inhibitory action on motoneurones indicate that the same transmitter substance is concerned with all. Since the inhibitory interneurones appear to lie entirely within the grey matter, the inhibitory substance should be extractable from grey matter. So far no success has been achieved. Florey and McLennan (1955a,b) have reported that their factor I isolated from cerebral cortex has some of the properties that would be expected for the inhibitory transmitter substance, but the significance of these experiments is doubtful. In particular, the rapid blockage of tendon reflexes (within 5 sec.) by application of a solution of factor I to the dorsum of the spinal cord is much more likely to be due to a direct blocking action on the dorsal roots than to an inhibitory action directly exerted on motoneurones. Two samples of factor I, kindly provided by Dr. Florey, were found to have no effect on monosynaptic reflexes when tested by intra-arterial injection into the spinal cord (Curtis, Eccles, and Eccles, 1955). This negative result might be attributable to the failure of factor I to penetrate the blood-brain barrier.

Though pharmacological tests have indicated that various inhibitory actions on motoneurones are mediated by the same transmitter substance, it must not be assumed that there is only one inhibitory transmitter. Evidence for another transmitter is provided by the inhibition that is evoked by stimulation of the reticular formation and the cerebellum and which is not depressed by strychnine. For example, this inhibition is very effective against strychnine tetanus of the spinal cord even after very high dosages with strychnine (Bremer, 1953b; Gernandt and Terzuolo, 1955).

4. The Supply of Transmitter Substances

a. Depletion and replenishment

When a sympathetic ganglion is perfused with an eserinized medium (Locke's solution plus glucose, or diluted blood, or blood), and the presynaptic fibres are stimulated repetitively, the output of acetylcholine in the perfusate progressively declines from a high initial value (Brown and Feldberg, 1936; MacIntosh, 1938; Emmelin and MacIntosh, 1948, 1956; Perry, 1953). With the superior cervical ganglion of the cat, the initial output is as high as 10^{-10} g per volley (Feldberg and Vartiainen, 1934; Perry, 1953; Emmelin and MacIntosh, 1956), and it falls more rapidly and to a lower level the higher the frequency of stimulation. There is a corresponding decline in synaptic transmission. After about 30 minutes of continuous stimulation, the output has fallen to a low steady level of about 4×10^{-9}g *per minute,* regardless of the frequency of stimulation, which may be taken as the rate of production of the acetylcholine available for synaptic transmission (Brown and Feldberg, 1936; Perry, 1953). In contrast, the total acetylcholine content of the ganglion (about 2.5×10^{-7}g) is much less diminished even by prolonged preganglionic stimulation (Brown and Feldberg, 1936; Kahlson and MacIntosh, 1939). On cessation of stimulation, there is a very rapid replenishment of the total acetylcholine content of the ganglion (Kahlson and MacIntosh, 1939), but in contrast there is a slow recovery in the response to preganglionic volleys, the output of acetylcholine produced by a second test stimulation being still low after a rest period as long as 35 minutes.

In explanation of these observations, Perry (1953) has proposed that much of the extractable acetylcholine of the ganglion exists in a form that is not available for release by preganglionic impulses and is slowly converted into available acetylcholine. On the contrary, when there is no eserine in the perfusion fluid, synaptic transmission is well maintained even during prolonged stimulation (Brown and Feldberg, 1936). Under such conditions it is not possible to measure the liberation of acetylcholine, because destruction by the cholinesterase prevents its appearance in the perfusate. Its output can be tested when, after eserinization, a second similar preganglionic tetanus is applied. Under such conditions, after a rest period of only 10 minutes, the output is equivalent to that of the control ganglion during the initial response and far greater than for the second tetanus of the control ganglion. Thus, in the absence of eserine, there is a very effective replenishment of the acetylcholine available for liberation.

All the experimental observations can be explained by an hypothesis proposed by Perry (1953) and can be shown diagrammatically in Figure 75. It is assumed that the liberated acetylcholine can be used to synthesize available acetylcholine only when it is hydrolysed by cholinesterase.

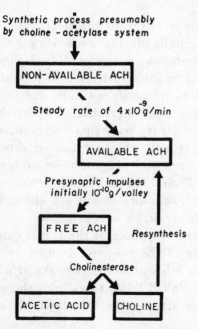

Synthetic process presumably by choline - acetylase system

NON-AVAILABLE ACH

Steady rate of 4×10^{-9} g/min

AVAILABLE ACH

Presynaptic impulses initially 10^{-10} g/volley

FREE ACH

Resynthesis

ACETIC ACID   CHOLINE

Cholinesterase

Figure 75

Diagram illustrating the postulated acetylcholine metabolism in cat superior cervical ganglion. Further explanation in text.

This mechanism will account for the maintenance of acetylcholine liberation during prolonged stimulation of a ganglion untreated by eserine. In addition, available acetylcholine is continually being formed at a slow steady rate of about 4×10^{-9}g per minute, presumably by some change in the nonavailable acetylcholine. The effect of choline in causing an increased output of acetylcholine and recovery of synaptic transmission (Brown and Feldberg, 1936) suggests that it is this product which is of special significance in replenishment of available acetylcholine. Perry further postulates that a presynaptic volley liberates a constant fraction of the available acetylcholine, a suggestion that was also made by Liley and North (1953) in their proposed explanation of post-tetanic potentiation.

It is possible that replenishment of acetylcholine also occurs by flow along the presynaptic fibres either of acetylcholine itself or of the choline-acetylase system, for MacIntosh (personal communication) finds that acetylcholine accumulates central to the severed end of a cholinergic nerve, the concentration attaining a value up to three times normal.

There has been no attempt to record the electrical responses of sympathetic ganglia during such very prolonged stimulations, but there was a considerable decline in synaptic transmission of impulses after a few seconds of repetitive stimulation, which was shown to be due to a depression of presynaptic action (Larrabee and Bronk, 1947). A decline of the excitatory postsynaptic potential was also observed to set in after the first two or three responses to a repetitive series of preganglionic volleys (J. C. Eccles, 1943; R. M. Eccles, 1955). Presumably these depressions of presynaptic excitatory action are attributable to the depletion of the available acetylcholine.

With monosynaptic reflex responses of the spinal cord there is a large depression of the response evoked by a second volley in the same afferent fibres (Brooks *et al.*, 1950b; Brock, Eccles, and Rall, 1951). It has been shown that this depression is not attributable to a lowering of motoneuronal responsiveness, hence it indicates a diminution in the presynaptic excitatory action, which presumably is due to a diminished output of transmitter substance, just as occurs with the sympathetic ganglion. A virtually complete recovery by 3 sec. was reported by Eccles and Rall (1951b) and by Jefferson and Schlapp (1953), but by a very precise technique Lloyd (1956) has found that a period of up to 20 sec. was required. The depression was observed to be cumulative during a repetitive series of postsynaptic potentials and to be more intense the faster the frequency (Eccles and Rall, 1951a). Depression to about 50 per cent was observed after about 10 responses at 400 a sec. Thus, so far as has been investigated, repetitive monosynaptic excitation of motoneurones results in a depression of presynaptic action, which parallels that of sympathetic ganglia and which likewise may be attributed to depletion of transmitter substance.

b. Mechanism of liberation
of transmitter substance from nerve terminals

The mechanism of liberation has been investigated in detail only with acetylcholine at the neuromuscular junction, but there is evidence that essentially the same mechanism is involved in the liberation of acetylcholine in sympathetic ganglia; hence it is possible that it obtains for other cholinergic junctions as well, e.g., for the action of motor-axon collaterals on Renshaw cells.

At the neuromuscular junction the nerve endings are responsible for evoking two kinds of depolarization of the postjunctional membrane: the end-plate potential produced by a nerve impulse, and the miniature end-plate potentials that occur spontaneously in a random manner (Fatt and Katz, 1952). By a pharmacological investigation it has been shown that both types of end-plate potential are produced by the liberation of acetylcholine from the nerve terminals. The miniature end-plate potentials are produced by quantal ejections of some thousands of molecules of acetylcholine from a multitude of foci over the surface of the nerve terminal. Each ejection is virtually independent of all other ejections. Normally the end-plate potential evoked by a nerve impulse is about 100 times larger than the miniature end-plate potentials. The end-plate potential can be greatly depressed, however, by soaking the preparation in a low-calcium Ringer solution in which some of the sodium had been replaced by magnesium (Castillo and Katz, 1954a,b,c; Liley, 1956b). Such depressed end-plate potentials are seen to be compounded of a very few units identical with the randomly occurring miniature end-plate potentials; hence it can be assumed that the nerve impulse produces an end-plate potential by the same quantal mechanism that is responsible for the miniature end-plate potentials. The arrival of an impulse at the nerve terminal causes an almost synchronous ejection of many quanta of acetylcholine, which otherwise could later have been ejected spontaneously to give the miniature end-plate potentials. Thus, the quantal mechanism accounts for both types of depolarization of the postjunctional membrane.

Depolarization of the nerve terminals by an extrinsically applied current greatly increases the frequency of miniature end-plate potentials (Castillo and Katz, 1954d; Liley, 1956b), while moderate hyperpolarization produces a decrease (Liley, 1956b). Probably the effect of raised potassium concentration in increasing the frequency of miniature end-plate potentials is also attributable to its depolarizing action on the nerve terminals (Liley, 1956c). Thus it may be postulated that all depolarizations of the nerve terminals activate the quantal ejection mechanism. The large and rapid potential change produced by the nerve impulse would be very potent in this respect, hence it evokes the large and virtually synchronous pile of ejected quanta that produces the end-plate potential. Furthermore, increase of the spike potential by anelectrotonic polarization causes a large increase in the end-plate potential (Castillo and Katz, 1954d). These various membrane depolarizations are effective in activating the quantal ejection mechanism, however, only if there is adequate calcium in the bathing fluid (Castillo and Katz, 1954a, b, and d; Brink, 1954; Liley, 1956b). At the optimal concentration of external calcium (about 10 mM to 20 mM), the end-plate potential of curarized muscle is increased about three fold above that observed at the normal level of calcium (Kuffler, 1944; Castillo and Stark, 1952), hence it may be concluded that the number of quanta contributing to the end-plate potential would be approximately three times the effective number under normal conditions, i.e., about 300. On the other hand, magnesium opposes this adjuvant action of calcium (Castillo and Engbaek, 1954; Castillo and Katz, 1954a), yet neither calcium nor magnesium significantly affects the frequency of miniature end-plate potentials (Fatt and Katz, 1952; Castillo and Katz, 1954a). Thus it has to be postulated (cf. Brink, 1954) that calcium and magnesium act on the process whereby depolarization of nerve terminals activates the quantal ejection mechanism, but not on the quantal ejection mechanism itself, as is illustrated in Figure 76.

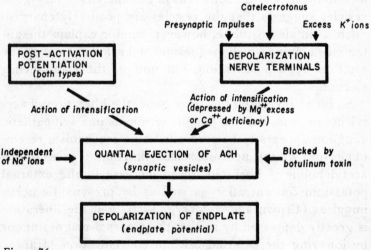

Figure 76

Diagram illustrating the factors which are believed to be operative in the ejection of acetylcholine from the presynaptic terminals of cholinergic fibres innervating striated muscle fibres or sympathetic ganglion cells. Further explanation in text.

Botulinum toxin has been shown to abolish the miniature end-plate potentials at about the same time as it
blocks neuromuscular transmission (Brooks, 1956). It
seems, therefore, that it has the unique ability to block
the quantal ejection mechanism and so block neuromuscular transmission. This contrasts with the curare type of
block where acetylcholine is still liberated in full amount,
but it has a diminished effectiveness on the subsynaptic
membrane.

Electron microscopy has revealed a likely histological
correlate of the quanta of acetylcholine (cf. Castillo and
Katz, 1955b). Small vesicles about 300 Å in diameter are
found in great numbers in the nerve terminals (cf. Figure 1C,E) and are clustered especially on the membrane
that is in contact with the muscle (Palade and Palay, 1954,
1956; Robertson, 1956; de Robertis and Bennett, 1955).
Some of these synaptic vesicles may even appear to have
burst on the surface. Such spontaneous bursting would
account for the miniature end-plate potentials. The effect of
membrane depolarization in causing an increased passage of
vesicles suggests that the vesicles are positively charged.
Such a simple postulate, however, cannot explain the antagonist actions which magnesium and calcium have on the
ejection by depolarization, but not on the spontaneous
ejection.

So far as investigations have gone, the liberation of acetylcholine from the presynaptic terminals in a sympathetic
ganglion appears to be controlled by a mechanism resembling that at the neuromuscular junction. For example,
acetylcholine is liberated by an increase in the external
potassium concentration as well as by presynaptic nerve
impulses (Brown and Feldberg, 1936) and the liberation
is greatly depressed by raising the external magnesium or
by lowering the external calcium concentration (Harvey
and MacIntosh, 1940; Hutter and Kostial, 1954; 1955). In
the absence of calcium, transmission is blocked (Bronk,
1939; Brink, Bronk, and Larrabee, 1946). Again the release of acetylcholine by nerve impulses or by potassium

is independent of the external sodium concentration (Hutter and Kostial, 1955), exactly as is indicated by the end-plate potential at the neuromuscular junction (Castillo and Katz, 1955b). The effect of depolarizing the presynaptic terminals does not yet seem to have been investigated, but on analogy with the neuromuscular junction it may be assumed that nerve impulses and potassium are effective in liberating acetylcholine because of the membrane depolarization that they produce (Hutter and Kostial, 1955), and further that external calcium is necessary for this liberation (Brink, 1954). So far intracellular recording has failed to reveal miniature synaptic potentials of ganglion cells (R. M. Eccles, 1956). Possibly they are too small to be detected above the noise level. Alternatively, there may be no background quantal ejection of acetylcholine from presynaptic terminals that are not depolarized. Again the synaptic vesicles in the presynaptic terminals (de Robertis and Bennett, 1955) probably play a key role in the manufacture and liberation of acetylcholine. The concentration of synaptic vesicles in the presynaptic terminals can be correlated with the finding that the concentration of transmitter substance (acetylcholine) in the preganglionic fibres within the ganglion is much higher than in the preganglionic nerve trunk (MacIntosh, personal communication).

When applied by direct injection, botulinum toxin blocks the cholinergic synaptic transmission from motor-axon collaterals to Renshaw cells (Brooks and Curtis, 1956). Presumably it does this, just as at the neuromuscular junction, by preventing the release of acetylcholine from the presynaptic terminals.

There is no other experimental evidence relating to the mechanism of liberation of acetylcholine or other transmitter substances at central synapses. All presynaptic terminals so far investigated, however, contain accumulations of synaptic vesicles (de Robertis and Bennett, 1955; Palade and Palay, 1954, 1956; Robertson, 1956) and such similar behaviour is exhibited by the various types of synapses that comparable mechanisms may be presumed. Of particular significance is the increased synaptic effectiveness that follows presynaptic activation, the so-called post-tetanic potentiation. "Postactivation potentiation," however, is a more appropriate term because some types of potentiation are observed after a single volley.

c. Postactivation potentiation

Following single or repetitive presynaptic impulses there is often potentiation of the postsynaptic response that is elicited by a test impulse in the same presynaptic fibre. The following criteria have been established in a series of investigations (Schaefer and Haass, 1939; Feng, 1941; Eccles, Katz, and Kuffler, 1941; Larrabee and Bronk, 1947; Lloyd, 1949; 1952b; Eccles and Rall, 1951b; Ström, 1951; Job and Lundberg, 1953; Liley and North, 1953; Jefferson and Benson, 1953; J. C. Eccles, 1953; Castillo and Katz, 1954c) and serve to distinguish between this class of phenomena and other conditions of increased response and facilitation.

(i) The potentiation is measured by an increased postsynaptic potential or by an increased postsynaptic discharge.

(ii) This potentiated response is elicited only by impulses in those presynaptic fibres that had been stimulated initially.

(iii) The potentiation is due to an increased presynaptic action, i.e., to an increased liberation of synaptic transmitter, and not to an increased excitability of the postsynaptic membrane.

There appears to be two different varieties of postactivation potentiation as so defined, the second type having a subvariety, which has been observed with the monosynaptic reflex during the first second after a brief high frequency conditioning tetanus, and which may be called "early postactivation potentiation" (Eccles and Rall, 1951b; Lloyd, 1952b).

First, there is the progressive increment of end-plate

potentials that is observed with repetitive stimulation of nerves to amphibian or crustacean muscles. It has been shown that the potentiated responses have an increased number of quantal components (Castillo and Katz, 1954c). This type of potentiation is distinguished from the other type because it is largest after very few stimuli and also because a maximum effect is produced by a testing impulse that immediately follows the conditioning impulse or impulses, and progressively less effect is observed with lengthening of the testing interval, so that at ordinary temperatures very little potentiation survives beyond 100 msec. (Feng, 1941; Eccles, Katz, and Kuffler, 1941). A further distinctive feature is revealed when rapid repetitive presynaptic impulses are employed as a test. There is a progressively increased response to the first few impulses, while an immediate and rapid decline occurs with the other type (cf. Figure 77B).

The principal type of postactivation potentiation has been observed at all junctional regions. It is characterized by the relatively slow phase of increment that follows the conditioning response and by a duration that, with the exception of the subvariety, extends for many seconds or even minutes. The mammalian sympathetic ganglion is exceptional in that a considerable potentiation follows a single conditioning volley (Larrabee and Bronk, 1947; Job and Lundberg, 1953). As with other junctions, much larger and more prolonged potentiations are built up by repetitive stimulation. The remarkable effectiveness of prolonged repetitive stimulation serves to distinguish this type of potentiation from the other type described above, in which two or three impulses have the maximum potentiating action, the end-plate potential being increased about three fold. For example, Feng (1941) found that the amphibian end-plate potential was potentiated very little after 200 impulses at 200/sec., whereas 4,000 and 12,000 impulses were, respectively, 20 and 40 times more effective. By making special postulates about the intensity and time course of an antagonistic depression, it would be possible

to maintain that all transitions exist between the two main
types of postactivation potentiation. It should be pointed
out, however, that additional postulates would also be
required to account for the time course of the subvariety,
early postactivation potentiation, and that part, at least, of
the principal type of postactivation potentiation is attributable to an increase in size of presynaptic nerve impulses
that is brought about by the hyperpolarization following
intense repetitive activity (Lloyd, 1949; Eccles and Rall,
1951b; Lloyd, 1952b).

Usually only a single stimulus has been employed in testing for postactivation potentiation. When repetitive presynaptic volleys have been employed for the testing stimulus, however, there has been a rapid decline in the
response to the successive volleys (Figure 77A,B), so that
there has been little or no potentiation after the first few
volleys (Ström, 1951; Eccles and Rall, unpublished observations; Liley and North, 1953). As shown by comparing
Figure 77B with the control (Figure 77A), the first EPSP
is potentiated by about 60 per cent and thereafter there is
a rapid decline of the potentiation so that it is less than
20 per cent with the sixth EPSP of the repetitive series.
Thus, this type of postactivation potentiation does not result from a large increase in the total amount of available
transmitter substance in the presynaptic terminals. There
appears rather to be an increase in the amount that is immediately available for liberation by the first few impulses
(Liley and North, 1953). It would be expected, therefore,
that little or no increase in the amount of liberated transmitter substance would be detectable in a perfusate, since
hundreds of volleys are required to liberate an amount
that is detectable experimentally. There appears to be no
report of such an investigation. It has invariably been
observed, however, that the potentiation is associated with
and attributable to an increase in the postsynaptic potential (EPSP or EPP) produced by a single testing presynaptic volley (Eccles and Rall, 1951b; R. M. Eccles,
1952a; Liley and North, 1953; J. C. Eccles, 1953), so an

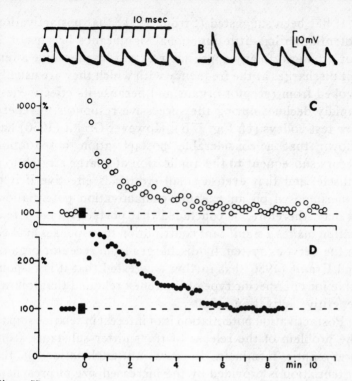

Figure 77

A, B. EPSP's recorded from a motoneurone in response to a repetitive monosynaptic excitation, 6 volleys at 45 per sec. Record B was taken at height of the postactivation potentiation that was induced by a prolonged high frequency stimulation of the testing afferent nerve, 600 per sec. for 15 sec. Record A is control response in the absence of potentiation (Curtis and Eccles, 1956). *C, D.* Effect of a burst of repetitive nerve stimulation on responses that are recorded intracellularly from a muscle fibre of rat diaphragm. The period of repetitive stimulation (200 per sec. for 15 sec.) is represented by a rectangular block, and time is measured from its cessation. *C.* Frequencies of miniature end-plate potentials measured as percentages of its initial control frequency of about 4 per sec. *D.* Sizes of end-plate potentials of a fibre curarized by soaking in 10^{-6} D-tubocurarine chloride and measured as percentages of the initial control value (Liley, 1956a).

increased output of transmitter substance may be presumed, especially as there is no associated increase in the response that is normally evoked when the transmitter is applied by perfusion (Larrabee and Bronk, 1947).

It has been suggested (Ström, 1951) that postactivation potentiation has little functional significance because it is not produced to any appreciable extent by repetitive afferent discharges at the frequency with which they are usually evoked from receptor organs and because its effectiveness rapidly declines during the successive responses to repetitive test volleys (cf. Fig. 77B). However Granit (1956) has shown that a considerable postactivation potentiation occurs subsequent to the application of a large stretch to a muscle, and that even a small stretch is effective if it is superimposed on an existing postactivation potentiation. It may, therefore, be concluded that postactivation potentiation makes a significant contribution to responses evoked in the nervous system by discharges from receptor organs, and Granit (1956) has further suggested that it is responsible for one specific type of the reflex rebound that follows repetitive activation.

Postactivation potentiation is of interest in relationship to the problem of the release of transmitter substance from presynaptic terminals. In part, an explanation of the potentiation is provided by the increased size of presynaptic spike that occurs during the after-hyperpolarization following activity (Lloyd, 1949, 1952a; Eccles and Rall, 1951b), for it has been demonstrated that an impulse causes a greater quantal release of transmitter substance from hyperpolarized nerve terminals (Castillo and Katz, 1954d). This explanation does not cover the whole duration of the postactivation potentiation (Eccles and Rall, 1951b; Liley and North, 1953), however, and under some conditions a large potentiation is associated with a diminished presynaptic spike. Furthermore, another change in the presynaptic endings has been found during postactivation potentiation at the mammalian neuromuscular junction. There is a great increase in the frequency of miniature end-plate potentials (Brooks, 1956; Liley, 1956a), which declines with the same time course as the potentiation of the end-plate potential evoked in a curarized muscle by a testing nerve impulse (Figure 77C,D). It differs in that it is largest immediately after the end of the conditioning tetanus, whereas the potentiation takes several seconds or even a minute to attain its maximum (Liley, 1956a).

It already has been postulated that miniature end-plate potentials are caused by the spontaneous bursting of synaptic vesicles, and that a presynaptic impulse momentarily causes a large intensification of this process. It can now be postulated that presynaptic impulses in addition cause a mobilization of synaptic vesicles so that the spontaneous release occurs at a higher frequency and more are discharged by a later testing presynaptic impulse. The delayed development of postactivation potentiation indicates that immediately after a tetanus a presynaptic impulse has diminished effectiveness in operating the quantal release mechanism, much as is observed when there is low calcium or high magnesium in the bathing fluid.

Since intense synaptic activation leads to the development of enhanced synaptic activity (miniature end-plate potentials as well as the end-plate or postsynaptic potentials), it is attractive to postulate that this is an example of functional compensation, depletion of the reserve supply of chemical transmitter leading to an excess replenishment of available transmitter. This postulate, however, receives no support from the finding that there is a rapid decline in the potentiation during a repetitive series of testing impulses (Figure 77B) so that after a few test impulses the potentiation may even give place to depression (cf. Liley and North, 1953). In conclusion, it can be stated that postactivation potentiation seems to be attributable to two events localized in the immediate region of the presynaptic membrane: a mobilization there of a relatively small number of synaptic vesicles, and an increased size of the presynaptic impulse.

CHAPTER VI

ASPECTS OF THE FUNCTIONAL ARCHITECTURE OF THE CENTRAL NERVOUS SYSTEM

A. THE CHEMICAL TRANSMISSION FROM A NERVE CELL

According to a principle first enunciated by Dale (1935), which may be called Dale's principle, any one class of nerve cells operates at all of its synapses by the same chemical transmission mechanism. This principle stems from the metabolic unity of a single cell, which extends to all of its branches. For example, the mitochondria of even the furthest axon terminals all derive ultimately from the same nucleus. An interesting example of this principle is provided by the motoneurone, which acts by the liberation of acetylcholine both at the motor endings of muscle fibres and at the synaptic endings of axon collaterals on Renshaw cells. Another interesting consequence is that according to Dale's principle the group Ia afferent fibres from muscle will be acting by the same excitatory transmitter substance at the synaptic endings which they make with three different classes of nerve cells: motoneurones, group Ia intermediate neurones, and the neurones of Clarke's column.

B. THE POSTSYNAPTIC ACTION OF A TRANSMITTER SUBSTANCE

It has been found that, in all the inhibitory pathways that have been investigated, the synaptic inhibitory action on motoneurones is exerted by short-axon interneurones. Conceivably the inhibition could be produced by the same transmitter substance that is responsible for excitatory synaptic transmission (cf. J. C. Eccles, 1953, pp. 171-73), specialization of the respective subsynaptic membranes accounting for the inhibitory or excitatory action, much as is presumed to occur with the opposite actions of acetylcholine (or adrenaline) on different smooth muscle fibres. It appears that this solution was not practicable in the morphogenesis of the central nervous system, where instead a change in the transmitter substance was secured by inserting a special interneurone even on the direct inhibitory pathway with all the consequential complications and the delay of an additional synaptic mechanism. It is, therefore, postulated that any one transmitter substance always has the same synaptic action, i.e., excitatory or inhibitory, at all synapses on nerve cells. According to this principle, any one class of nerve cells will function exclusively either in an excitatory or in an inhibitory capacity at all of its synaptic endings, i.e., there are functionally just two types of nerve cells, excitatory and inhibitory. The Renshaw cells, the group Ia intermediate neurones, and the other intermediate neurones on the inhibitory pathways for group Ib and cutaneous impulses would be examples of neurones that were exclusively inhibitory in function, and which consequently may be termed "inhibitory neurones." On the other hand, the dorsal root ganglion cells with their primary afferent fibres, probably the neurones of all the long tracts both ascending and descending, the motoneurones, and many interneurones belong to the class of "excitatory neurones." Conceptually, by this subdivision of nerve cells into excitatory and inhibitory types, a great simplification is produced in the physiology of central synaptic mechanisms, for all branches of any one neurone can be regarded as having the same synaptic function, i.e., as being uniformly excitatory or uniformly inhibitory.

In attempting to understand the operation of any neuronal system in the central nervous system of vertebrates, a useful provisional postulate would be that all inhibitory cells are short-axon neurones lying in the grey matter, while all transmission pathways including the peripheral afferent and efferent pathways are formed by the axons of excitatory cells. Such a postulate would be of most direct application in relation to such simple problems as the modes of termination of the descending tracts, but eventually it may be also applicable to more complex situations in the brain stem and even in the cerebellar and cerebral cortices. In all these situations there is as yet no information on the structural features of the inhibitory mechanisms.

C. THE DURATION OF ACTION OF
TRANSMITTER SUBSTANCES

According to the above two principles there is identity of transmitter substance and of transmitter action at all of the synapses made by one class of neurone. There may, however, be considerable divergences in the duration of transmitter action. For example, the duration of the effective transmitter action exerted by a group Ia volley on motoneurones is so brief (cf. Figure 11A) that a single volley never sets up more than one discharge from motoneurones, and this also seems to occur with the action of such a volley on the cells of Clarke's column (Laporte, Lundberg, and Oscarsson, 1956), while this same volley causes a transmitter action which is prolonged enough to set up a repetitive discharge from some group Ia intermediate neurones (cf. Figure 59C–E). A particularly long duration of transmitter action is exhibited by the cholinergic activation of Renshaw cells, where a single volley may cause a transmitter action that is as long as 3 sec. when the cholinesterase has been inactivated (Figure 65D). A relatively long action is also seen with the activation of intermediate neurones by group Ib or cutaneous afferent volleys (Figure 70A–C), and with the activation by cutaneous volleys of neurones discharging up the dorsal spinocerebellar tract (Figure 70L). With all these diverse synapses, however, the latency of the synaptic action is of about the same duration (0.3 msec. to 0.5 msec.) when measured from the time of arrival of the presynaptic volley to the onset of the postsynaptic response.

Evidence has already been presented for an extraordinarily long duration (several seconds) of the transmitter action on the ganglion cells of *Aplysia,* and for a long action (about 20 msec.) by the inhibitory transmitter on crustacean stretch receptor cells. With the sympathetic ganglion the synaptic transmitter, acetylcholine, also had an effective duration of 10 msec. to 20 msec.

It can be calculated that, if the transmitter substance is free to diffuse and has approximately the diffusion coefficient of acetylcholine, it will diffuse away so rapidly from a focus of the dimensions of a synapse that its concentration will have fallen to a negligible level within 1 msec. of its liberation (Fatt, 1954; Ogston, 1955). When the cholinesterase is inactivated, the acetylcholine transmitter action on Renshaw cells declines at a rate that is thousands of times slower than the calculated free diffusional rate. This decline is progressive from the maximum that is attained within 1 msec. It seems, therefore, that there must be some barrier, as illustrated in Figure 78, that restrains the diffusion of acetylcholine away from the synapse. Since the duration of transmitter action is much briefer (about 50 msec.) when the cholinesterase is active (cf. Figures 64B,D,G; 65A), the cholinesterase must be located within the barrier (cf. Figure 78). With a parasympathetic ganglion, Szentágothai, Donhoffer, and Rajkovits (1955) have found the cholinesterase to be associated with both the presynaptic and postsynaptic surfaces of the synapses.

The effectiveness of cholinesterase in shortening the duration of the transmitter action indicates that the prolonged action (about 3 sec.) is not susceptible to an alter-

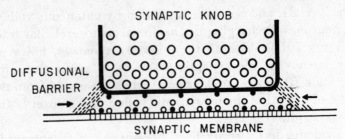

Figure 78

Diagram showing the postulated barrier that impedes the diffusion of acetylcholine from the synaptic regions of Renshaw cells. Acetylcholine is indicated by open circles, cholinesterase by filled circles, and the acetylcholine receptor surface by the striated border on the subsynaptic membrane.

native explanation, namely, that the acetylcholine adheres for this long time to the receptor areas of the subsynaptic membrane. Possibly the diffusional barrier also accounts in part for the relative ineffectiveness of intra-arterially injected acetylcholine in stimulating Renshaw cells (cf. Figure 65).

The concept of a diffusional barrier around synapses may account for the considerable duration of transmitter action of cutaneous impulses on interneurones (Figure 70A,B,C) and on the neurones discharging up the dorsal spinocerebellar tract (Figure 70L). This barrier would be far less effective, however, than that for synapses on Renshaw cells. Barriers having a comparable degree of permeability presumably account for the relatively long transmitter actions exerted by inhibitory impulses on the crustacean stretch receptor cells and by excitatory impulses on sympathetic ganglion cells.

A diffusional barrier around synapses would increase the effectiveness of synaptic transmitter action, as is required for example in the concept of "effective synaptic space" (Emmelin and MacIntosh, 1956), and also prolong the duration of temporal facilitation. This latter effect would be of particular importance in the activation of Renshaw cells by the relatively slow frequency motoneuronal discharges, which are usually below 50 per sec. There is as yet no structural correlate for these postulated diffusional barriers, but possibly it may be the close glial investment of synapses (Wyckoff and Young, 1956). Possibly also the ground substance described by Hess (1953, 1955) may contribute to the formation of diffusional barriers.

D. THE STRUCTURAL FEATURES OF A SYNAPSE

The synapse has been defined as the synaptic knob, the subsynaptic membrane, and the synaptic cleft of about 200 Å that lies between them (cf. Figure 1D,E). The significant features for present purposes are the area of the synaptic contact and the width of the cleft. Essentially the synapse is a device for applying minute amounts of a specific chemical substance to the special receptor area of the subsynaptic membrane, which in turn becomes highly permeable to some or all ions. The resulting electric current flows through the synaptic cleft and so to the remainder of the postsynaptic membrane, including that of the initial segment (cf. Figure 11A). Thus there are two conflicting requirements in regard to the width of the synaptic cleft: that it should be very narrow, so that the synaptic transmitter is applied as efficiently and as quickly as possible to the subsynaptic membrane; that it should be wide, so that the postsynaptic currents flow as freely as possible.

The first requirement would be satisfied by a cleft only 200 Å in width, for the diffusion time across it would be about 1 μsec. By making certain probable assumptions, it is possible to show that the second requirement is also likely to be satisfied by a cleft of 200 Å. The high conductance of the activated subsynaptic membrane (up to 2×10^{-6} mhos. for the monosynaptic synapses) indicates that the subsynaptic membrane of any one synapse has a very high specific conductance. For example, it would be as high as 0.2 mho/cm^2 if the total area of the activated subsynaptic membrane was 10^{-5} cm^2. This estimate is in reasonable agreement with the estimate of 0.25 mho/cm^2 for the maximum conductance of the end-plate membrane while it is generating the end-plate potential (Fatt and Katz, 1951; Castillo and Katz, 1954e; Eccles, 1953, p. 86). If the specific resistance of the fluid in the synaptic cleft is 100 Ωcm, which is rather higher than for an ultrafiltrate of blood, it can be calculated that with a synaptic knob 2 μ in diameter the resistance offered to current flow through the cleft is effectively only about 3 per cent of that offered in its passage through the subsynaptic membrane. Thus, there seems an adequate safety margin for the efficient operation of the cleft in carrying current to the whole subsynaptic membrane. For example, it is possible that glial structures in and around the cleft might significantly raise the specific resistivity above the 100 Ωcm that has been assumed. However, even if this occurred by a factor of five, the cleft would still have an adequate conductance. Presumably the accurate setting of the cleft width is dependent on some structural organization in the cleft, but, if it were of lattice or sponge construction, e.g., a gel formation, the resistance should not be greatly raised.

If the area of the synaptic contact was considerably increased, e.g., to 10 μ in diameter, the cleft resistance would be so greatly increased relative to the membrane resistance that the synaptic mechanism would become inefficient in evoking the flow of postsynaptic currents. A sufficient area of synaptic contact is thus more efficiently secured by having many small synapses than a few very large synapses. However, large club-like synaptic endings up to 10 μ in diameter occur in the central nervous systems of some animals (Bodian, 1937; 1942; 1952; Horstmann, 1954). Of particular interest are the giant synapses on the cells of Clarke's column in the cat spinal cord. The areas of apparent synaptic contact are very elongated, being hundreds of microns long, but only a few microns across (Szentágothai and Albert, 1955), a design which would minimize the resistance presented by the synaptic cleft. Finally these giant synaptic contacts terminate in large end bulbs up to 15 μ by 8 μ in size. The width of the synaptic cleft must be known before the mode of operation and the efficiency of these various types of large synapse can be appreciated.

It can be concluded that the synaptic knob of about 2 μ in diameter separated by a cleft space of about 200 Å from the subsynaptic membrane is a structure that is very effectively designed for efficient synaptic transmission of either excitatory or inhibitory actions. Any one presynaptic fibre can secure a sufficient area of synaptic contact by branching so that it has many synaptic knobs on the same neurone (cf. Cajal, 1909; 1934; Lorente de Nó, 1938; Bodian, 1942; Chang, 1952).

E. THE POSSIBLE SIEVE-LIKE STRUCTURE OF THE SUBSYNAPTIC MEMBRANE

It has been shown that all experimental investigations on the mode of production of the EPSP and the IPSP of motoneurones are sufficiently explained by postulating that presynaptic impulses cause brief increases in the ionic permeability of the respective subsynaptic membranes: to all ions with the EPSP (Chapter II); and with the IPSP only to such small hydrated ions as K^+ and Cl^-, Na^+ in particular being excluded (Chapter III). Thus we may envisage the respective subsynaptic membranes as being converted momentarily into a sieve-like structure as is schematically illustrated in Figure 79, the pore sizes of the excitatory membrane being large enough to allow all of the tested ions to pass, while with the inhibitory membrane the pore sizes are small enough to account for the selective permeability, SCN^- ions being the largest that penetrate freely, while Na^+ ions are excluded. It is not suggested that the actual pores in the membrane have these sizes. It can merely be stated that this is the effective size so far as the passage of ions is concerned. It is of further interest

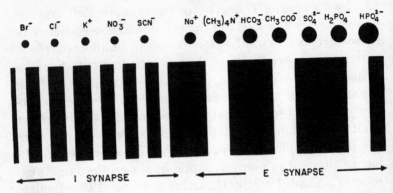

SIZES OF HYDRATED IONS

Figure 79

Schematic representation of the postulated sieve-like structure of the sub-synaptic membranes of an inhibitory and an excitatory synapse when under the influence of the appropriate transmitter substance. The effective pores of the inhibitory synapse are shown large enough to admit all hydrated ions in the series from Br^- to SCN^-, while excluding all others shown in the diagram. The effective pores of the excitatory synapses are large enough to admit all the ions. The filled circles show the relative diameters of the hydrated ions as derived from the limiting ionic conductances on the assumption that the ions are spherical.

that the positive or negative charge on the ion appears to have no influence on its ability to pass through the pores, though, of course, the potential gradient across the membrane affects the passage of charged particles in the manner expected from theoretical considerations (Coombs *et al.*, 1955b).

It already has been pointed out that the conclusions regarding the ionic permeabilities of the subsynaptic membranes of motoneurones are in good agreement with observations on other postjunctional membranes. For example, there is good evidence that with amphibian muscle the end-plate potential is generated because the end-plate membrane becomes permeable to all ions (Fatt and Katz, 1951; Castillo and Katz, 1954e). On the other hand, the inhibitory responses at a variety of junctions, crustacean stretch receptor cells, crustacean neuromuscular junctions, and vagal junctions in cardiac muscle, are probably produced by a selective permeability to the small ions, K^+ and Cl^-, Na^+ ions being largely excluded.

Thus, at all junctional regions that have been investigated sufficiently, the transmitter substance appears to operate by converting the postjunctional (subsynaptic) membrane to a sieve-like structure, the pores being much larger with excitatory than with inhibitory junctions. The passage of any ion species through the pores would depend only on the size of the hydrated ion, being independent of its charge or of its chemical nature. In contrast, very specific chemical criteria govern the ionic permeabilities during and after the impulse (cf. Huxley, 1954), which can be regarded as the response of the membrane to an electric excitation that causes a sufficient depolarization. Thus, during the rising phases of the spikes of nerve and muscle fibres, there is a specific increase in the permeability to Na^+ ions only (Hodgkin, 1951; Hodgkin and Huxley, 1952b,c), the single known exception being indicated by the imperfect substitution of some quaternary ammonium ions with the B fibres of amphibian nerves (Lorente de Nó, 1949). Likewise, during the falling phase of the spike and the after-hyperpolarizations that follow, there is an increased permeability to K^+ ions alone (Hodgkin, 1951; Hodgkin and Huxley, 1952b,c; Coombs *et al.*, 1955a), though Rb^+ ions might be a possible substitute for K^+ ions (Hodgkin, 1947).

It is possible to show that these differences in the ionic permeability mechanisms of the surface membranes result in increased efficiency both in the production of the impulse and in the transmitter mechanisms. Thus, the large specific permeability to Na^+ ions causes the impulse to generate a higher voltage with a consequent increased rate of propagation, while the subsequent increase in K^+ ion permeability accelerates the recovery of the membrane potential so that it is ready to propagate another impulse. It appears that the specific increase in Na^+ ion permeability cannot be initiated by a chemical transmitter mechanism. On the other hand, by making the subsynaptic membrane permeable to all ions, the excitatory transmitter is able to generate a much larger depolarizing current than would be produced if the same membrane area became specifically sodium permeable, as during a spike. For example, with the amphibian end-plate membrane the density of the inward currents during the end-plate potential may be as large as $3 \times 10^{-2} A/cm^2$, while during the steepest rising phase of the spike it is only about $3 \times 10^{-3} A/cm^2$ (cf. Eccles, 1953, p. 78). Similarly in generating the EPSP of motoneurones the density of the current across the subsynaptic membrane is considerably larger than that occurring across the membrane generally during the rising phase of the SD spike. Conceivably a synaptic inhibitory action could be produced by a specific increase in permeability to K^+ ions only, but again the outward current through the subsynaptic membrane would be much lower than that produced by the increased permeability to all small ions.

Reference already has been made in Chapter II to the possibility that a loss of responsiveness of the subsynaptic membrane to electrical stimuli may be a consequence of its specialized reaction to chemical transmitter substances. Probably the most striking example is seen in the slow muscle fibres of amphibian muscle. Impulses in the small motor fibres evoke the small-nerve junctional potentials which involve the whole length of a slow muscle fibre and never lead on to a spike potential (Kuffler and Vaughan Williams, 1953). In fact, depolarization of the surface membrane by an electrical current, no matter how intense, never evokes a propagated spike potential or even a local response (Burke and Ginsborg, 1955). The surface membrane appears to be devoid of the sodium permeability mechanism that produces the rising phase of a spike potential (Hodgkin and Huxley, 1952c). The electric organs of Torpedo and the ray resemble these amphibian slow muscle fibres in responding to the chemical transmitter from nerve impulses but not to electrical stimulation (Fessard, 1946; 1952; Fessard and Posternak, 1950; Albe-Fessard, 1951; Brock, Eccles, and Keynes, 1953).

F. THE DENDRITIC STRUCTURE

On both anatomical and physiological grounds the dendrites of motoneurones become of progressively less significance for the purposes of synaptic function the further they extend from the soma. The density of synaptic knobs falls off progressively (Lorente de Nó, 1938; Barr, 1939; Bodian, 1952; Wyckoff and Young, 1956), and the increased electrotonic decrement causes the postsynaptic currents generated by activation of a synapse to have progressively less effect on the membrane potential of the initial segment of the axon, which is the site of the effective excitatory and inhibitory actions of synapses, at least with motoneurones. It has been calculated that the length constant for a standard dendrite is about 300 μ, so it will be appreciated that synapses on dendrites are virtually ineffective if situated on the more remote regions of dendrites that are about 1 mm in length. Possibly the ineffectiveness of the more distally located synapses is a factor that has contributed morphogenetically to secure this sparse distribution.

The long apical dendrites of the cortical pyramidal cells are particularly suitable for an investigation of dendritic properties, because of both their length and their orientation in parallel. The simplest situation occurs in the Ammon's horn, where the pyramidal cells occur in a single layer with the apical dendrites oriented perpendicular thereto (Lorente de Nó, 1934). By employing extracellular recording with a penetrating microelectrode, Cragg and Hamlyn (1955) have shown that synaptic stimulation of the apical dendrites evokes a slow depolarization having much the same duration (about 15 msec.) as the monosynaptic EPSP of motoneurones, thus confirming and adding to the observations of Renshaw, Forbes, and Morison (1940). If this depolarization is large enough, there may be superimposed on it a spike potential of 1 msec. to 3 msec. in duration, which propagates very slowly (about 0.4 metres per sec.) down to the soma. With activation of pyramidal cells in the somatic region, propagation out along the apical dendrites also was observed and had the same velocity. Thus, it seems that apical dendrites differ from the dendrites of motoneurones in that impulses are generated in them by synaptic excitatory action. Morphologically, too, they are different, being essentially an extended part of the soma and having a dense coverage by synaptic knobs all along their length (Cajal, 1934; Chang, 1952). Since the apical dendrites are 600μ to 700μ in length and only about 3μ in diameter, there would probably be a negligible electrotonic transmission from their apical terminals to the soma, as is also indicated by the very slow conduction velocity for impulses. The generation of impulses in peripheral areas of apical dendrites, however, ensures that no functional disability results from this negligible electrotonic transmission. It appears that there are several relatively independent synaptic fields at different levels on the apical dendrites and on the soma with its basal dendrites. Probably this also occurs with the Mauthner cell, where very different synaptic structures are seen at different locations (Bodian, 1937; 1940; 1942; 1952).

In many respects the apical dendrites of pyramidal cells in other areas of the cerebral cortex give responses similar to those of the Ammon's horn. There has been a general tendency to distinguish sharply between the locations of the slow and fast potentials, the former being regarded as arising in the dendrites, the latter being produced in the somas and axons (Jung, 1953a; Bishop and Clare, 1953; Clare and Bishop, 1955a,b; Chang, 1955). A similar differentiation was proposed by Tasaki, Hagiwara, and Watanabe (1954) for the Mauthner cell. This distinction between the origins of the two potentials is supported by the usual experimental observation that synaptic, antidromic, and direct excitatory actions fail to evoke spike potentials in the superficial regions of the cortex, where there are no somas or axons of pyramidal cells, but only dendrites. In lightly anaesthetized preparations, however, brief spikes of about 1 msec. in duration have been recorded there (Amassian, 1953; Li and Jasper, 1953). Possibly such spikes are usually too small to appear above the background noise and also they may be suppressed by too deep an anaesthesia (cf. Chang, 1955). On the other hand, all investigators record from that region slow potentials of about 10 msec. in duration, and there is now good evidence that such potentials are produced by synaptic action, being essentially EPSP's (Jung, 1953b; Li and Jasper, 1953; Cragg and Hamlyn, 1955; Perl and Whitlock, 1955). Chang (1955) argues against this conclusion because he finds that a slow potential (about 10 msec. in duration) is generated in response to an antidromic volley propagating up from the pyramidal tract. It has been shown, however, that, when antidromic impulses fail to invade crustacean stretch receptor cells, they evoke slow polarizing responses which resemble EPSP's (Eyzaguirre and Kuffler, 1955b). As suggested in the discussion on Figure 33C–E, the depolarized cell has to restore its membrane potential, exactly as occurs after the active depolarizing phase of the EPSP.

It has been suggested that the postsynaptic potential is propagated only electrotonically from the apical dendrite to the soma (Jung, 1953a; Clare and Bishop, 1955a,b). The very slow conduction velocity for impulse propagation along the apical dendrites of pyramidal cells (about 0.2 to 0.6 metres per sec., Chang, 1955) indicates that there would be a very large decrement in the electrotonic transmission from the distal regions of the dendrite to the soma. Thus it seems likely that, just as with the pyramidal cells of the Ammon's horn, the synaptic excitatory actions on the more distal regions of the apical dendrites become effective largely by generating impulses which propagate to the soma and axon (cf. Amassian, 1953; Li and Jasper, 1953).

Sholl (1953) has studied in detail the size and arrangement of the dendrites of cortical neurones, and their opportunities for synaptic contact. With the pyramidal cells, the apical dendritic system has been treated as a zone separate from that of the basal dendrites. With each of these zones, relatively few dendrites extend beyond 200 μ from the focal points, which are, respectively, the soma and the main bifurcation of the apical dendrite. Up to such distances the electrotonic spread of EPSP's would be reasonably effective, so these two zones could function as separate convergence centres with the independent ability to generate impulses. Possibly there is another zone along the apical shaft, for it is very richly covered by synaptic endings (Chang, 1952). Because of these relatively independent zones for the initiation of impulses, the pyramidal cell would be expected to have a more complex behaviour than a motoneurone. Intracellular recording (cf. Figure 31) provides an experimental method for testing these various suggestions.

With the motoneurone, synaptic stimulation appears never to be effective in initiating impulses in dendrites. Intracellular recording reveals that impulses always commence in the initial axonal segment (cf. Figures 14, 15, 19). The question thus arises: what function, if any, is subserved by the terminal regions of the motoneuronal dendrites with all their profuse branches? Consideration of the ionic exchanges between a motoneurone and its environment shows that, with normal continuous activity, it is likely to be embarrassed by the progressive increase of sodium and depletion of potassium. For example, with a standard motoneurone it has been estimated that each impulse will entail an intake of about 5 to 10 x 10^{-15} equiv. of Na$^+$ ions and a loss of the same amount of K$^+$ ions. Motoneurones can be stimulated to discharge at a frequency as high as 50 a sec. for considerable periods (Adrian and Bronk, 1929; Barron and Matthews, 1938), which would entail a gain of at least 15 p. mole of Na$^+$ ions per minute and a loss of 15 p. mole of K$^+$ ions. The maximum rate at which Na$^+$ ions can be pumped outward has been given as about 10 p. mole per minute, so it is evident that under such conditions the motoneurone would be steadily gaining in sodium and losing potassium, with the result that in a few minutes it would have the same abnormal ionic composition and would give the same disordered responses as the motoneurones of Figures 26, 37B, and 38B. Such responses could be regarded as an example of fatigue. A possible safeguard against an excessive development of this fatigue effect could be provided by the dendrites. Even under resting conditions impulses propagate very slowly (about 1 metre per sec.) up the dendrites of motoneurones (Lorente de Nó, 1953; Fatt, 1956a), much as occurs with the apical dendrites of pyramidal cells, and there is evidence that propagation ceases before the terminals (Barakan *et al.*, 1949), which indicates a very low safety factor for propagation. This safety factor would be lowered progressively as the sodium increased and the potassium decreased during prolonged activity; hence successive impulses would leave more and more of the dendrites uninvaded. Thus, there would be a progressive falling off in the ionic exchanges during the spikes, and the whole dendritic surface would still be available for pumping sodium outward and potassium inward. In this way the dendrites would provide a safety device operating with a time scale of minutes and tending to limit the increase in sodium and loss of potassium during activity that is prolonged over many minutes. Under such conditions there would be a diffusional flow of sodium from soma up the dendrites and of potassium in the reverse direction.

G. INTERNEURONES AS COMMON PATHS

Because of the methods of experiment that have been employed in studying the simpler reactions of the nervous system, undue emphasis has been placed on investigations of motoneurones, because their responses are so readily recorded in ventral roots and peripheral nerves. As a consequence, the concepts of convergence and of the final common path have been developed almost exclusively for motoneurones.

By employing a microelectrode for extracellular recording, the responses of interneurones can be investigated
readily. Observations such as those illustrated in Figures 59A–C and 60 reveal that several different afferent
fibres of the same type converge onto an intermediate neurone, and this is also readily demonstrable with Renshaw
cells (cf. Figure 64B). In addition, convergence occurs for
fibres of different sensory modalities. As shown in Figure 61, a group Ia intermediate neurone is excited to discharge impulses, not only by the group Ia impulses of a
muscle group, but also by group III afferent impulses of
diverse muscles and by a wide variety of cutaneous impulses. It thus acts as a common path for the inhibitory
action which all these various modalities exert on the
antagonist group of motoneurones. Similarly, it is found
that Renshaw cells may be excited by group III muscle
impulses and by cutaneous impulses and thus also act as a
common path for inhibitory action. Presumably a more
impressive convergence onto interneurones would be demonstrable if volleys were also set up in descending tracts
(cf. Lloyd, 1941a,c; Lloyd, 1942; Niemer and Magoun,
1947; Lloyd and McIntyre, 1948; Szentágothai, 1951). In
addition to the converging excitatory paths on interneurones, it is possible at times to demonstrate converging
inhibitory impulses in the high threshold group III fibres
of both cutaneous and muscle nerves (Figure 80). It was
postulated above that the action of strychnine and tetanus
toxin in potentiating polysynaptic reflexes was due to depression of such interneuronal inhibition.

Much more investigation on interneurones is required
before their responses are as well documented as those
of motoneurones (cf. Bernhard, 1952a). There is sufficient
information, however, to show that interneurones play an
important role as convergence centres for diverse types of
afferent impulses, and hence relieve motoneurones from
the full burden of integrative activity at the level of the
spinal cord. We may surmise that integration likewise
occurs at all levels of the central nervous system. Work

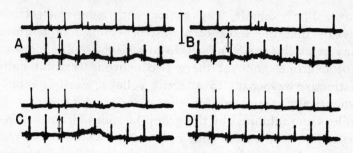

Figure 80

Upper records are spike responses of an intermediate neurone to repetitive volleys in the group Ia fibres of the quadriceps nerve at 220 per sec., the lower records giving spike responses in the L6 dorsal root (cf. Figure 59 D–F). In *A, B,* and *C,* the double arrow signals a single stimulus setting up a biceps-semitendinosus volley, the stimulus strengths being approximately 2, 4, and 10 times threshold. *D* gives control response to the repetitive quadriceps stimulation alone. Potential scale indicates 5 mV for the intermediate cell responses (Eccles, Fatt, and Landgren, unpublished observations).

on the responses of single cells already has given many examples in the cells of the cerebral cortex, of the reticular formation, of the thalamus, and of various other nuclei in the brain stem and spinal cord (Amassian, 1952; Rose and Mountcastle, 1954; Tasaki, Polley, and Orrego, 1954; Laporte, Lundberg, and Oscarsson, 1956; Davies, Berman, and Mountcastle, 1955; Jung, Baumgarten, and Baumgartner, 1952; Galambos, Rose, Bromily, and Hughes, 1952; Galambos, 1952; Amassian, and DeVito, 1954; Jung, and Baumgartner, 1955; Baumgartner, 1955; Scheibel, Scheibel, Mollica, and Moruzzi, 1955).

H. CHEMICAL TRANSMITTERS AND SPECIFICITY OF SYNAPTIC CONNECTIONS

One of the most perplexing problems in the organization of the nervous system arises because of the specificity of synaptic action on neurones that have overlapping dendritic fields (cf. Romanes, 1953, and the ensuing discussion). For example, exploration with a microelectrode reveals that the soma of a gastrocnemius motoneurone may be as close as 50 μ to 100 μ to a biceps-semitendinosus motoneurone, and yet these two neurones exhibit quite distinctive responses to afferent volleys. Each is mono-synaptically activated by the corresponding group Ia volleys and inhibited by the group Ia volleys from antagonists. The dendrites of such cells may be as much as 1 mm long, so there is a large overlap of the dendritic fields and there is overlap even of the large dendritic branches on which effective synaptic action would be exerted. Possibly the selective synaptic connections were established before the large dendritic outgrowth. Possibly, too, aberrant synaptic connections on remote parts of the dendrites would not produce detectable potentials in the soma or appreciably modify the generation of impulses in the initial segment of the axon. This latter suggestion is supported by the many occasions when aberrant monosynaptic excitatory connections have been observed, as, for example, a biceps-semitendinosus motoneurone that is monosynaptically excited by group I afferent impulses from both gastrocnemius and biceps-semitendinosus muscles. (Eccles, Eccles, and Lundberg, unpublished observations.) Thus, it is conceivable that each synergic group of motoneurones may be sufficiently discrete from other groups to account for the observed degree of specificity of its reflex response.

In some nuclei the soma and dendrites of neurones are very compactly arranged so that the specificity of operation is readily explicable on such anatomical grounds, as, for example, the cells of Clarke's column (cf. Cajal, 1909, Figure 117), of the inferior olive (Scheibel and Scheibel, 1955), and of the lateral geniculate body. In this latter situation the branches of several presynaptic fibres make a feltwork enclosing six to eight cells, so forming the cellular glomerulus of Taboada (1927), which appears to be a functional unit for that synaptic relay (cf. Bishop, 1953). Of particular significance is the attempt which Scheibel and Scheibel (1955) have made to utilize their detailed anatomical knowledge in an attempt to understand the mode of operation of the inferior olive. The profuse yet compact dendritic trees of the olivary cells and the large interpenetration between adjacent dendritic trees provide a structure with most interesting potentialities for co-ordination of the various afferent inflows (cf. Grundfest and Carter, 1954).

However, neurones may be in very close apposition and yet exhibit distinctive responses to afferent inputs, i.e., the closest juxtaposition of neurones need not result in identity of functional synaptic connections thereon. For example, systematic exploration by a microelectrode reveals that the large and small motoneurones of a muscle are interspersed within the motor nucleus of that muscle (cf. Eccles, 1955, Figure 3E), and yet at least in one respect very different synaptic connections are made upon them. Small motoneurones exhibit no trace of the powerful monosynaptic excitatory action which is exerted on large motoneurones by group Ia impulses of that muscle or its synergists (Hunt, 1951; Eldred, Granit, and Merton, 1953; Granit, 1955). In other respects very extensive investigations have shown that there is a fairly close parallelism between the responses of the small and large motoneurones of a synergic group of muscles, the former differing merely in their lower threshold of activation (Hunt, 1951; Granit and Kaada, 1952; Eldred, Granit, and Merton, 1953; Eldred and Hagbarth, 1954; Granit, 1955). It would appear that the selective action of group Ia impulses provides the only enigma, for on purely anatomical grounds the small motoneurones should also be supplied with synaptic articulations from the group Ia fibres. It seems necessary, therefore, to invoke a chemical specificity and to postulate that small motoneurones are not sensitive to the transmitting substance liberated from group Ia afferent fibres. As first suggested by Dale (1935), a chemical specificity of this type would account for the failure of many cross-union experiments in the peripheral nervous system to establish functional connections.

The chemical specificity of transmitting substances is also of interest in connection with the neurones that are serially arranged in the pathways of the central nervous system. The question arises: Is any regularity observable in the sequences of transmitter substances? In a study of the choline-acetylase content of the successive links in such chains of neurones, Feldberg and Vogt (1948) found that there was evidence of alternation between neurones that effectively manufactured acetylcholine, i.e., contained a choline-acetylase system, and hence presumably were cholinergic in their synaptic action, and neurones that lacked this property. For example, in accordance with this generalization, the primary afferent fibres of somaesthetic sensation are not cholinergic, the secondary afferent fibres arising from the cuneate and gracile nuclei are probably cholinergic, and, finally, the tertiary afferent fibres arising from the lateral thalamic nucleus would again not be cholinergic (cf. Feldberg, 1954). Likewise on the optic pathway there is evidence of cholinergic transmission in the retina from bipolar cells to retinal ganglion cells (Hebb, Silver, Swan, and Walsh, 1953; Francis, 1953), while the optic nerve fibres are not cholinergic excitors of lateral geniculate neurones, though these in turn appear to be cholinergic (cf. Feldberg, 1954). Much more investigation of these various synaptic mechanisms, however, is required before their cholinergic nature can be regarded as established. As already suggested, nicotine and dihydro-β-erythroidine are two drugs that are likely to give significant results in this respect. Finally, as Feldberg (1954) points out, one situation appears to be contrary to the alternation hypothesis. Preganglionic parasympathetic fibres act cholinergically on ganglion cells (Perry and Talesnik, 1953), which in turn are believed to act cholinergically on their peripheral effector organs. The interesting implications of the alternation hypothesis have been discussed by Jung (1953a).

So far the existence of inhibitory synaptic action has largely been ignored in the construction of diagrammatic representations of pathways in the higher levels of the central nervous system. It is evident that in an inhibitory pathway running through a chain of neurones there will be transmission by excitatory transmitter substances at all synapses until that of the final inhibitory neurones, where there is a change over to inhibitory transmitting substance. The actions of strychnine and of tetanus toxin, particularly when given by local injection, should aid in the detection of such inhibitory neurones.

I. THE PLASTICITY REACTIONS OF NERVE CELLS

Under this general heading there is a wide variety of very slow changes in both the structure and the physiological behaviour of nerve cells. Reference may be made to Jung (1953a) and J. C. Eccles (1953) for a more complete account. For the most part our information about these changes is fragmentary and a major task for the future is to extend and organize this information so that functional changes may be explained in terms of the structural alterations. Hitherto the briefer functional changes that occur with synaptic facilitatory and inhibitory reactions have been explained by membrane changes which would not be detectable even by electron microscopy. Even the more prolonged changes of postactivation potentiation would be expected to be associated merely with a small increase in the density of synaptic vesicles just inside the presynaptic membrane. On the contrary, a wide variety of structural changes have been found to occur when the axons of neurones are severed (the axon-reaction or chromatolysis) or even when neurones suffer from disuse, transneuronal degeneration being perhaps a special example of this, and from over-usage.

After the axon of a nerve cell is severed, there is a sequence of changes that leads eventually to complete recovery after many weeks. Within a few days the Nissl

substance virtually disappears and the nucleus moves
excentrically, while the protein content falls to a very low
value owing apparently to a transient depression of protein synthesis (Hydén, 1943). A relationship of Nissl substance to protein synthesis has also been suggested by
Palay and Palade (1955). At a later stage the growth of
the regenerating axon causes a serious drain on the protein
manufacturing apparatus of the nucleus, which becomes
intensely active (Hydén, 1943). Concurrently there are
large changes in the responses of the neurones to synaptic
excitation, but so far no correlation of structural and functional change has been possible. For example, Brown and
Pascoe (1954) find that, some days after section of a postganglionic sympathetic trunk, there is almost complete
failure of synaptic transmission through the ganglion.
They have shown further that under such conditions preganglionic volleys evoke a normal output of acetylcholine,
and that the blockage is probably due to a diminished
sensitivity of the ganglion cells to acetylcholine. A suggested explanation is that the observed diminution of
cholinesterase (McLennan, 1954) has caused the accumulation of acetylcholine with a consequent blocking action
due to depolarization. Though such blockage is produced
when cholinesterase is inactivated, it is difficult to see how
the observed halving of cholinesterase activity could result
in a depolarization adequate for this purpose. It should also
be stated, however, that the blockage does not seem explicable by any of the demonstrable structural changes.

Likewise the changed responses of motoneurones after
section of their axons cannot be related to the structural
changes. As with the sympathetic ganglion, the monosynaptic excitatory action is greatly depressed, though it
is not known whether or not this is due to a lowered effectiveness of the transmitter substance. Whatever the explanation, the usual monosynaptic reflexes cannot be
elicited for several weeks. Thereafter a slow recovery
ensues, though it is still incomplete after nine weeks
(Downman, Eccles, and McIntyre, 1953). Concurrent with

the depressed monosynaptic activity of group I impulses, there is a great development of reflex discharges having much longer synaptic delays (1.5 msec. to 5 msec.), though still evoked by group I impulses from muscle. There is also an increase in the polysynaptic reflex responses from cutaneous nerve volleys. These effects regress after several weeks with return of the normal monosynaptic activity. On the basis of intracellular recording, Bradley, Brock, and McIntyre (1955) recently have proposed that the responses to the group I afferent volleys have longer synaptic actions because the monosynaptically evoked EPSP exhibits a rising phase which has a lower slope, but a greatly prolonged duration. It is doubtful if their experiments have excluded the possibility that in part this prolongation is due to polysynaptic excitatory action. In any case, no structural correlate has been discovered for these remarkable functional changes. For example, Barr (1940) could detect no change in the synaptic knobs on chromatolysed cells. It seems likely, however, that changes will be revealed by the more refined technique of electron microscopy. Downman et al., (1953) suggested that the chromatolysing neurones released a chemical evocator which caused the sprouting and growth of neighbouring nerve fibres and so led to the development of the polysynaptic reflexes.

Growth processes controlled by evocators from degenerating neurones have been postulated under other circumstances (cf. below). Histological investigation has revealed the outgrowths of nerve fibres so evoked, and similarly should be employed to determine whether there are fibre outgrowths that could be responsible for the delayed synaptic responses of chromatolysed motoneurones.

A depression of monosynaptic excitatory action also was found some weeks after the afferent nerve fibres had been severed just peripheral to the dorsal root ganglia (Eccles and McIntyre, 1953). In part, at least, this could be explained by the observed small shrinkage of the dorsal root fibres (Eccles and McIntyre, 1953; Szentágothai and

Rajkovits, 1955). The monosynaptic reflexes, however, exhibited two abnormal features which could not be explained by a mere deficiency of synaptic excitatory action. A conditioning tetanus was followed by a large postactivation potentiation which ran a time course several times slower than normal and which declined to a level of reflex activity much higher than the initial controls. This residual potentiation persisted for hours after a few minutes of tetanization; hence it has been concluded that this intense period of usage is compensating temporarily for the deleterious effect which the long period of disuse had on synaptic function. Presumably the synaptic deficiency would arise in part because of the shrinkage of the synaptic knobs. Such a shrinkage has been observed after some months of a disuse that was brought about by removal of the long bones of a limb, the nerve trunks being untouched (Szentágothai and Rajkovits, 1955). But the abnormal course of postactivation potentiation suggests that in addition, disuse may cause a disability in the manufacture and availability of transmitter substance.

If disuse thus has a deleterious effect on the excitatory potency of synapses, it follows that normal usage has a sustaining function, and it is further likely that excess usage will lead to an enhancement of the normal excitatory potency. Unfortunately, the experimental data is very meagre and there is only fragmentary evidence in support of this important inference. For example, increased monosynaptic reflexes were observed in the segment adjacent to the operatively inactivated segments (Eccles and McIntyre, 1953), and functionally overloaded muscles were found to have hypertrophied nerve fibres (Edds, 1950). If these observations can be substantiated and extended, it appears that we have here at the simplest reflex level synaptic behaviour which could form the basis of conditioned reflexes and learning phenomena for more complex regions of the central nervous system (cf. J. C. Eccles, 1953, pp. 216-27).

Physiologists have been too ready to assume that in

mammals the structural pattern of the nervous system has been fixed very early in life and that subsequently no re-adjustments are possible. Doubtless this attitude stems from the almost complete failure of experiments on functional regeneration after section of the mammalian spinal cord (cf. Scott and Clemente, 1955). Furthermore, experiments on cross-union of nerves and muscle transplantation in general have failed to demonstrate functional readjustments of mammalian reflexes, as is revealed by the comprehensive and critical review by Sperry (1945). It could be maintained, however, that these experiments had not been sufficiently subtle either in their operative procedures or in their subsequent experimental testing. Certainly an operative lesion of the central nervous system is followed by a great outgrowth of nerve fibres (cf. Cajal, 1928). Thus, it is generally agreed that the regenerative failure is not due to a lack of regrowth, but rather to a misdirection of the regenerating fibres, which occurs particularly because of the large development of glial and fibrous tissue at the site of the lesion.

In some recent experiments it has appeared that, given more favourable situations, nerve fibres in the mammalian central nervous system can be stimulated to grow and achieve new functional connections (McCouch, Austin, and Liu, 1955; Magladery and Teasdale, 1956). For example it is found that some weeks or months after hemisection of the spinal cord an afferent volley produces cord potentials and polysynaptic reflex responses which are larger than those produced by a similar volley on the control side. Possible effects from higher centres were eliminated by complete transection of the cord at the start of the final experimental investigation. Under these conditions it appears that chemical evocators are produced by the degenerating fibres of the ventrolateral tracts and these cause the observed outgrowth of branches from adjacent nerve fibres, e.g., of the short propriospinal tracts. It is presumed that these branches establish functional connections much as has been postulated with nerve fibres adjacent to chromatolysing motoneurones (Downman *et al.*, 1953). Such an effect of degenerating nerve fibres would be of great significance in relation to compensatory reactions following clinical lesions of the nervous system.

Remarkable regenerative power is exhibited by the spinal cord of teleostean fish (Kirsche, 1950) and the amphibian nervous system also displays a very great plasticity (cf. Weiss, 1952; Sperry, 1951). For example, a normal behaviour pattern is exhibited eventually by a transplanted amphibian limb. It does not seem possible to develop an explanation of such remarkable effects which conforms with orthodox neurophysiological concepts (cf. Weiss, 1952). More intensive analytical investigation of reflex patterns is necessary before the theoretical implications can be appreciated, but at least it seems that new and important concepts will be required. Special reference should be made to the attempt by Sperry (1951) to develop the concept of specification, but it seems that a much deeper understanding of the factors controlling growth and the establishment of functional connections is required before adequate hypotheses can be formulated. We may conclude that the functional picture of a nerve cell which has been outlined in this monograph is deficient in so far as it fails to account for the plastic and developmental phenomena.

REFERENCES

[Numbers in square brackets at end of each entry indicate the pages on which it is cited.]

Adrian, E. D., and Bronk, D. W. (1929). The discharge of impulses in motor nerve fibres; Part II, The frequency of discharge in reflex and voluntary contractions. *J. Physiol.,* **67:** 119–51. [66, 226]

Adrian, R. H. (1956). The effect of internal and external potassium concentration on the membrane potential of frog muscle. *J. Physiol.,* **133:** 631–58. [9, 19]

Alanis, J. (1953). Effects of direct current on motor neurones. *J. Physiol.,* **120:** 569–78. [66]

——, and Matthews, B. H. C. (1952). The mechano-receptor properties of central neurones. *J. Physiol.,* **117:** 59–60P. [13]

Albe-Fessard, D. (1951). Modifications de l'activité des organes électriques par des courants d'origine extérieure. *Arch. Sci. Physiol.,* **5:** 45–73. [52, 222]

——, and Buser, P. (1954). Analyse microphysiologique de la transmission réflexe au niveau du lobe électrique de la torpille (Torpedo marmorata). *J. Physiologie,* **46:** 923–46. [8, 13, 93]

——, —— (1955). Activités intracellulaires recueillies dans le cortex sigmoïde du Chat: Participation des neurones pyramidaux au "potentiel evoque" somesthesique. *J. Physiologie,* **47:** 67–69. [85]

Alexandrowicz, J. S. (1951). Muscle receptor organs in the abdomen of *Homarus vulgaris* and *Palinurus vulgaris. Quart. J. micr. Sci.,* **92:** 163–99. [7, 88, 128]

—— (1952). Receptor elements in the thoracic muscles of *Homarus vulgaris* and *Palinurus vulgaris. Quart. J. micr. Sci.,* **93:** 315–46. [7, 88, 128]

Alvord, E. C., and Fuortes, M. G. F. (1953). Reflex activity of extensor motor units following muscular afferent excitation. *J. Physiol.,* **122:** 302–21. [66]

Amassian, V. E. (1952). Interaction in the somatovisceral projection system. *Res. Publ. Ass. nerv. ment. Dis.,* **30:** 371–402. [229]

—— (1953). Evoked single cortical unit activity in the somatic sensory areas. *Electroenceph. clin. Neurophysiol.,* **5:** 415-38. [225]

——, and DeVito, J. L. (1956). Transmission through the cuneate nucleus; a single unit analysis of a primary somatosensory relay. In press. [85, 176]

——, and DeVito, R. V. (1954). Unit activity in reticular formation and nearby structures. *J. Neurophysiol.,* **17:** 575–603. [229]

Amin, A. H.; Crawford, T. B. B.; and Gaddum, J. H. (1954). The distribution of substance P and 5-hydroxytryptamine in the central nervous system of the dog. *J. Physiol.,* **126:** 596–618. [191, 192]

Araki, T., and Otani, T. (1955). Response of single motoneurones to direct stimulation in toad's spinal cord. *J. Neurophysiol.,* **18**: 472–85. [8, 13, 16, 18, 19, 22, 30, 41, 46, 48, 50, 53, 55, 58, 69]

——, ——, and Furukawa, T. (1953). The electrical activities of single motoneurones in toad's spinal cord, recorded with intracellular electrodes. *Jap. J. Physiol.,* **3**: 254–67. [8, 13, 40, 53, 77]

Armstrong, D.; Dry, R. M. L.; Keele, C. A.; and Markham, J. W. (1953). Observations on chemical excitants of cutaneous pain in man. *J. Physiol.,* **120**: 326–51. [189]

Arvanitaki, A., and Chalazonitis, N. (1955). Potentiels d'activite du soma neuronique geant *(Aplysia). Arch. Sci. physiol.,* **9**: 115–44. [6, 7, 8, 13]

Austin, G. M. (1952). Suprabulbar mechanisms of facilitation and inhibition of cord reflexes. *Res. Publ. Assoc. nerv. ment. Dis.,* **30**: 196–222. [180]

Balthasar, K. (1952). Morphologie der spinalen Tibialis- und Peronaeus-Kerne bei der Katze: Topographie, Architektonik, Axon- und Dendritenenverlauf der Motoneurone und Zwischenneurone in den Segmenten L6-S2. *Arch. Psychiatr. und Zeits. Neurol.,* **188**: 345–78. [6]

Barakan, T. H.; Downman, C. B. B.; and Eccles, J. C. (1949). Electric potentials generated by antidromic volleys in quadriceps and hamstring motoneurones. *J. Neurophysiol.,* **12**: 393–424. [50, 227]

Barcroft, J. (1938). *Features in the Architecture of Physiological Function.* Cambridge University Press. [viii]

Barr, M. L. (1939). Some observations on the morphology of the synapse in the cat's spinal cord. *J. Anat.,* **74**: 1–11. [4, 52, 55, 223]

—— (1940). Axon reaction in motoneurones and its effect upon the end-bulbs of Held-Auerbach. *Anat Rec.,* **77**: 367–74. [235]

Barron, D. H., and Matthews, B. H. C. (1938). The interpretation of potential changes in the spinal cord. *J. Physiol.,* **92**: 276–321. [39, 66, 226]

Baumgartner, G. (1955). Reaktionen einzelner Neurone im optischen Cortex der Katze nach Lichtblitzen. *Pflüg. Arch. ges. Physiol.,* **261**: 457–69. [229]

Bernhard, C. G. (1952a). Reflex patterns in internuncial systems. *Res. Publ. Ass. nerv. ment. Dis.,* **30**: 68–86. [228]

—— (1952b). The cord dorsum potentials in relation to peripheral source of afferent stimulation. *Cold Spr. Harb. Symp. quant. Biol.,* **17**: 221–32. [38]

—— (1953). The spinal cord potentials in leads from the cord dorsum in relation to peripheral source of afferent stimulation. *Acta physiol. scand.,* **29**: Suppl. 106, 1–29. [38]

——; Bohm, E.; and Petersen, I. (1953). Investigations on the organization of the corticospinal system in monkeys. *Acta physiol. scand.,* **29**: Suppl. 106, 79–105. [178]

——, and Skoglund, C. R. (1953). Potential changes in spinal cord following extra-arterial administration of adrenaline and noradrenaline as compared with acetylcholine effects. *Acta physiol. scand.,* **29**: Suppl. 106, 435–54. [192]

——; Taverner, D.; and Widen, L. (1951). Differences in the action of tubocurarine and strychnine on the spinal reflex excitability of the cat. *Brit. J. Pharmacol.,* **6**: 551–59. [188]

Bishop, G. H., and Clare, H. (1953). Responses of cortex to direct electrical stimuli applied at different depths. *J. Neurophysiol.,* **16**: 1–19. [224]

——, and O'Leary, J. L. (1940). Electrical activity of the lateral geniculate of cats following optic nerve stimuli. *J. Neurophysiol.*, **3**: 308–22. [177]

———, ——— (1942). Factors determining the form of the potential record in the vicinity of the synapses of the dorsal nucleus of the lateral geniculate body. *J. cell. comp. Physiol.*, **19**: 315–31. [177]

Bishop, P. O. (1953). Synaptic transmission. An analysis of the electrical activity of the lateral geniculate nucleus in the cat after optic nerve stimulation. *Proc. Roy. Soc.*, B, **141**: 362–92. [55, 177, 230]

———; Jeremy, D.; and McLeod, J. G. (1953). Phenomenon of repetitive firing in lateral geniculate of cat. *J. Neurophysiol.*, **16**: 437–47. [177]

———, and McLeod, J. G. (1954). Nature of potentials associated with synaptic transmission in lateral geniculate of cat. *J. Neurophysiol.*, **17**: 387–414. [177]

Bodian, D. (1937). The structure of the vertebrate synapse. A study of the axon endings on Mauthner's cell and neighboring centers in the goldfish. *J. comp. Neurol.*, **68**: 117–59. [4, 218, 224]

——— (1940). Further notes of the vertebrate synapse. *J. comp. Neurol.*, **73**: 323, 343. [4, 224]

——— (1942). Cytological aspects of synaptic function. *Physiol. Rev.*, **22**: 146–69. [4, 218, 219, 224]

——— (1952). Introductory survey of neurons. *Cold Spr. Harb. Symp. quant. Biol.*, **17**: 1–13. [4, 55, 218, 223, 224]

Boyd, I. A., and Martin, A. R. (1956). Personal communication. [15]

Bradley, K.; Brock, L. G.; and McIntyre, A. K. (1955). Effects of axon section on motoneurone function. *Proc. Univ. Otago Med. Sch.*, **33**: 14–16. [235]

———; Easton, D. M.; and Eccles, J. C. (1953). An investigation of primary or direct inhibition. *J. Physiol.*, **122**: 474–88. [134, 135, 143, 144, 154, 188, 193]

———, and Eccles, J. C. (1953). Analysis of the fast afferent impulses from thigh muscles. *J. Physiol.*, **122**: 462–73. [99, 171]

Bremer, F. (1944). Le mode d'action de la strychnine à la lumière de travaux récents. *Arch. int. Pharmacodyn.*, **69**: 249–64. [188]

——— (1951). Aspects electrophysiologiques de la transmission synaptique. *Arch. int. Physiol.*, **59**: 588–602. [39, 180]

——— (1953a) *Some Problems in Neurophysiology*. University of London, The Athlone Press. [39, 186]

——— (1953b). Strychnine tetanus of the spinal cord. In: *The Spinal Cord*, 78–83. *Ciba Found. Symp.*, London: Churchill. [198]

———; Bonnet, V.; and Moldaver, J. (1942). Contribution à l'étude de la physiologie générale des centres nerveux. I. La summation centrale. *Arch. int. Physiol.*, **52**: 1–56. [39]

Brink, F. (1954). The role of calcium ions in neural processes. *Pharmacol. Rev.*, **6**: 243–98. [203, 205]

———; Bronk, D. W.; and Larrabee, M. G. (1946). Chemical excitation of nerve. *Ann. N. Y. Acad. Sci.*, **47**: 457–85. [204]

Brock, L. G.; Coombs, J. S.; and Eccles, J. C. (1952a). The recording of potentials from motoneurones with an intracellular electrode. *J. Physiol.*, **117**: 431–60. [7, 10, 12, 37, 39, 40, 48, 66, 69, 75, 77, 97, 180, 181]

———; ———; ——— (1952b). The nature of the monosynaptic excitatory and inhibitory processes in the spinal cord. *Proc. Roy. Soc.,* B, **140:** 170–76. [21, 32, 154]

———; ———; ——— (1953). Intracellular recording from antidromically activated motoneurones. *J. Physiol.,* **122:** 429–61. [7, 40, 48, 49, 51, 52]

———; Eccles, J. C.; and Rall, W. (1951). Experimental investigations on the afferent fibres from muscle nerves. *Proc. Roy. Soc.,* B, **138:** 453–75. [68, 200]

———; Eccles, R. M.; and Keynes, R. D. (1953). The discharge of individual electroplates in *Raia clavata. J. Physiol.,* **122:** 4–6P. [52, 222]

Bronk, D. W. (1939). Synaptic mechanisms in sympathetic ganglia. *J. Neurophysiol.,* **2:** 380–401. [182, 204]

Brooks, C. McC.; Downman, C. B. B.; and Eccles, J. C. (1950a). After-potentials and excitability of spinal motoneurones following antidromic activation. *J. Neurophysiol.,* **13:** 9–38. [82]

———; ———; ——— (1950b). After-potentials and excitability of spinal motoneurones following orthodromic activation. *J. Neurophysiol.,* **13:** 157–76. [68, 200]

———, and Eccles, J. C. (1947a). An electrical hypothesis of central inhibition. *Nature,* Lond., **159:** 760–64. [181]

———, ——— (1947b). Electrical investigation of the monosynaptic pathway through the spinal cord. *J. Neurophysiol.,* **10:** 251–74. [37, 39, 67]

———, ——— (1948). Inhibitory action on a motor nucleus and synaptic pathway through the spinal cord. *J. Neurophysiol.,* **11:** 401–16. [97]

———; ———; and Malcolm, J. L. (1948). Synaptic potentials of inhibited motoneurones. *J. Neurophysiol.,* **11:** 417–30. [148]

———, and Fuortes, M. G. F. (1952). Potential changes in spinal cord following administration of strychnine. *J. Neurophysiol.,* **15:** 257–67. [188]

Brooks, V. B. (1956). An intracellular study of the action of repetitive nerve volleys and of botulinum toxin on miniature end-plate potentials. *J. Physiol.* In press. [197, 204, 210]

———, and Curtis, D. R. (1956). Personal communication. [205]

———; ———; and Eccles, J. C. (1955). Mode of action of tetanus toxin. *Nature,* Lond., **175:** 120–21. [195, 196]

Brown, G. L. (1937). Transmission at nerve endings by acetylcholine. *Physiol. Rev.,* **17:** 485–513. [182]

———, and Feldberg, W. (1936). The acetylcholine metabolism of a sympathetic ganglion. *J. Physiol.,* **88:** 265–83. [198, 199, 200, 204]

———, and Gray, J. A. B. (1948). Some effects of nicotine-like substances and their relation to sensory nerve endings. *J. Physiol.,* **107:** 306–17. [189]

———, and Pascoe, J. E. (1954). The effect of degenerative section of ganglionic axons on transmission through the ganglion. *J. Physiol.,* **123:** 565–73. [234]

Buchthal, F.; Engbaek, L.; Sten-Knudsen, O.; and Thomasen, E. (1947). Application of adenosinetriphosphate and related compounds to the spinal cord of the cat. *J. Physiol.* **106:** 3–4P. [190]

Bulbring, Edith, and Burn, J. H. (1941). Observations bearing on synaptic transmission by acetylcholine in the spinal cord. *J. Physiol.,* **100:** 337–68. [184]

Bullock, T. H. (1948). Properties of a single synapse in the stellate ganglion of squid. *J. Neurophysiol.,* **11:** 343–64. [91, 92]

———, and Hagiwara, S. (1956). Personal communication. [91, 92, 94, 180]

Burgen, A. S. V., and Chipman, L. M. (1951). Cholinesterase and succinic dehydrogenase in the central nervous system of the dog. *J. Physiol.*, **114**: 296–305. [187]

———, and Terroux, K. G. (1953). On the negative inotropic effect in the cat's auricle. *J. Physiol.*, **120**: 449–64. [118, 152]

Burke, W., and Ginsborg, B. L. (1955). Membrane changes responsible for the small-nerve junctional potential. *J. Physiol.*, **129**: 9–10P. [52, 222]

Cajal, S. R. (1909). *Histologie du Système Nerveux de l'homme et des vertébrés*. Vol. I. Paris, Maloine. [153, 158, 161, 162, 176, 219, 230]

——— (1928). *Degeneration and Regeneration of the Nervous System.* Trans., R. M. May. London, Oxford Univ. Press. [237]

——— (1934). Les preuves objectives de l'unité anatomique des cellules nerveuses. *Trab. Lab. Invest. biol. Univ. Madr.*, **29**: 1–137. [1, 219, 224]

——— (1954). Neuron Theory or Reticular Theory? Trans. M. U. Purkiss and C. A. Fox. Madrid, Instituto "Ramon y Cajal." [1]

Caldwell, P. C. (1955). Studies of ionic mobilities in the giant axon of the squid by means of an intracellular electrode system. *J. Physiol.*, **129**: 16P. [23, 122]

del Castillo, J., and Engbaek, L. (1954). The nature of the neuromuscular block produced by magnesium. *J. Physiol.*, **124**: 370–84. [203]

———, and Katz, B. (1954a). The effect of magnesium on the activity of motor nerve endings. *J. Physiol.*, **124**: 553–59. [202, 203]

———, ——— (1954b). Quantal components of the end-plate potential. *J. Physiol.*, **124**: 560–73. [202, 203]

———, ——— (1954c). Statistical factors involved in neuromuscular facilitation and depression. *J. Physiol.*, **124**: 574–85. [202, 206, 207]

———, ——— (1954d). Changes in end-plate activity produced by presynaptic polarization. *J. Physiol.*, **124**: 586–604. [202, 210]

———, ——— (1954e). The membrane change produced by the neuromuscular transmitter. *J. Physiol.*, **125**: 546–65. [5, 58, 218, 220]

———, ——— (1955a). On the localization of acetylcholine receptors. *J. Physiol.*, **128**: 157–81. [5]

———, ——— (1955b). Local activity at a depolarized nerve-muscle junction. *J. Physiol.*, **128**: 396–411. [204, 205]

———, ——— (1955c). Effects of vagal and sympathetic nerve impulses on the membrane potential of the frog's heart. *J. Physiol.*, **129**: 48–49P. [98, 152]

———, and Stark, L. (1952). The effect of calcium ions on the motor end-plate potential. *J. Physiol.*, **116**: 507–15. [203]

Chang, H. T. (1952). Cortical and spinal neurons. Cortical neurons with particular reference to the apical dendrites. *Cold Spr. Harb. Symp. quant. Biol.*, **17**: 189–202. [52, 219, 224, 226]

——— (1955). Cortical response to stimulation of medullary pyramid in rabbit. *J. Neurophysiol.*, **18**: 332–52. [224, 225]

Chu, L. W. (1954). A cytological study of anterior horn cells isolated from human spinal cord. *J. comp. Neurol.*, **100**: 381–413. [2, 5, 7, 50, 52]

Clare, M. H., and Bishop, G. H. (1955a). Properties of dendrites; apical dendrites of the cat cortex. *EEG Clin. Neurophysiol.*, **7**: 85–98. [224, 225]

———, ——— (1955b). Dendritic circuits: the properties of cortical paths involving dendrites. *Amer. J. Psychiat.,* **111:** 818–25. [224, 225]

Cole, K. S., and Curtis, H. J. (1939). Electric impedance of the squid giant axon during activity. *J. gen. Physiol.,* **22:** 649–70. [23, 45, 77]

——, —— (1941). Membrane potential of the squid axon during current flow. *J. gen. Physiol.,* 24: 551–63. [15, 17]

Coombs, J. S.; Curtis, D. R.; and Eccles, J. C. (1956a). Time courses of motoneuronal responses. *Nature,* 178: 1049–50. [18, 19, 20, 32, 33, 35, 36]

——; ——; —— (1956b). The generation of impulses by motoneurones. In press. [39, 40, 41, 46, 49, 50, 53, 54, 66]

——; ——; and Landgren, S. (1956). Spinal cord potentials generated by impulses in muscle and cutaneous afferent fibres. *J. Neurophysiol.,* **19:** 452–67. [173, 179]

——; Eccles, J. C.; and Fatt, P. (1955a). The electrical properties of the motoneurone membrane. *J. Physiol.,* 130: 291–325. [6, 8, 10, 12, 13, 14, 15, 16, 17, 42, 43, 47, 48, 52, 71, 73, 75, 77, 79, 80, 81, 96, 126, 221]

——; ——; —— (1955b). The specific ionic conductances and the ionic movements across the motoneuronal membrane that produce the inhibitory post-synaptic potential. *J. Physiol.,* 130: 326–73. [8, 9, 10, 13, 23, 45, 81, 97, 104, 105, 106, 107, 108, 110, 113, 114, 115, 117, 119, 122, 123, 124, 125, 146, 220]

——; ——; —— (1955c). Excitatory synaptic action in motoneurones. *J. Physiol.,* 130: 374–95. [8, 21, 31, 33, 35, 39, 55, 57, 59, 60, 62, 63, 65, 181]

——; ——; —— (1955d). The inhibitory suppression of reflex discharges from motoneurones. *J. Physiol.,* 130: 396–413. [8, 21, 97, 100, 102, 135, 136, 137, 139, 141, 145, 147, 194]

Cragg, B. G., and Hamlyn, L. H. (1955). Action potentials of the pyramidal neurones in the hippocampus of the rabbit. *J. Physiol.,* 129: 608–27. [56, 223, 225]

Curtis, D. R., and Eccles, J. C. (1956). Unpublished observations. [209]

——; —— and Eccles, R. M. (1955). Pharmacological studies on reflexes. *Amer. J. Physiol.,* 183: 606. [184, 185, 189, 197]

Dale, H. H. (1935). Pharmacology and nerve endings. *Proc. R. Soc. Med.,* 28: 319–32. [163, 182, 190, 212, 231]

—— (1937). Transmission of nervous effects by acetylcholine. *Harvey Lectures,* 32: 229–45. [182]

Davies, P. W.; Berman, A. L.; and Mountcastle, V. B. (1955). A functional analysis of the first somatic area of the cat's cerebral cortex in terms of the activity of single neurons. *Amer. J. Physiol.,* 183: 607. [229]

Davson, H. (1952). *A Textbook of General Physiology.* London: Churchill. [118]

Denny-Brown, D. (1929). On the nature of postural reflexes. *Proc. Roy. Soc.,* B, 104: 253–301. [66]

Downman, C. B. B.; Eccles, J. C.; and McIntyre, A. K. (1953). Functional changes in chromatolysed motoneurones. *J. comp. Neurol.,* 98: 9–36. [234, 235, 238]

Eccles, J. C. (1936a). The actions of antidromic impulses on ganglion cells. *J. Physiol.,* 88: 1–39. [132]

—— (1936b). Synaptic and neuro-muscular transmission. *Ergebn. Physiol.,* 38: 339–444. [182]

—— (1943). Synaptic potentials and transmission in sympathetic ganglion.

J. Physiol., **101**: 465–83. [200]

—— (1946a). Synaptic potentials of motoneurones. *J. Neurophysiol.,* **9**: 87–120. [39]

—— (1946b). An electrical hypothesis of synaptic and neuromuscular transmission. *Ann. N. Y. Acad. Sci.,* **47**: 429–55. [181]

—— (1948). Conduction and synaptic transmission in the nervous system. *Ann. Rev. Physiol.,* **10**: 93–116. [186]

—— (1950). The responses of motoneurones. *Brit. med. Bull.,* **6**: 304–11. [37, 50]

—— (1952). The electrophysiological properties of the motoneurone. *Cold Spr. Harb. Symp. quant. Biol.,* **17**: 175–83. [21]

—— (1953). *The Neurophysiological Basis of Mind: The Principles of Neurophysiology.* Oxford, Clarendon Press. [viii, 30, 33, 138, 154, 183, 206, 208, 213, 218, 222, 233, 236]

—— (1955). The central action of antidromic impulses in motor nerve fibres. *Pflüg. Arch. ges. Physiol.,* **260**: 385–415. [47, 48, 49, 83, 231]

——; Eccles, R. M.; and Fatt, P. (1956). Pharmacological investigations on a central synapse operated by acetylcholine. *J. Physiol.,* **131**: 154–69. [163, 165]

——; Fatt, P.; and Koketsu, K. (1954). Cholinergic and inhibitory synapses in a pathway from motor-axon collaterals to motoneurones. *J. Physiol.,* **126**: 524–62. [76, 84, 98, 163, 165, 166, 168, 169, 194]

——; ——; and Landgren, S. (1956). The central pathway for the direct inhibitory action of impulses in the largest afferent nerve fibres to muscle. *J. Neurophysiol.,* **19**: 75–98. [98, 100, 154, 155, 156, 157, 158, 159, 161]

——; ——; ——; and Winsbury, G. J. (1954). Spinal cord potentials generated by volley in the large muscle afferents. *J. Physiol.,* **125**: 590–606. [37, 38, 160, 171]

——; Katz, B.; and Kuffler, S. W. (1941). Nature of the 'end-plate potential' in curarized muscle. *J. Neurophysiol.* **4**: 362–87. [206, 207]

——, and McIntyre, A. K. (1953). The effects of disuse and of activity on mammalian spinal reflexes. *J. Physiol.,* **121**: 492–516. [235, 236]

——, and Pritchard, J. J. (1937). The action potential of motoneurones. *J. Physiol.,* **89**: 43–45P. [82]

——, and Rall, W. (1951a). Repetitive monosynaptic activation of motoneurones. *Proc. Roy. Soc.,* B, **138**: 475–98. [201]

——, —— (1951b). Effects induced in a monosynaptic reflex path by its activation. *J. Neurophysiol.,* **14**: 353–76. [68, 201, 206, 208, 210]

Eccles, R. M. (1952a). Action potentials of isolated mammalian sympathetic ganglia. *J. Physiol.,* **117**: 181–95. [208]

—— (1952b). Responses of isolated curarized sympathetic ganglia. *J. Physiol.,* **117**: 196–217. [131, 183, 184]

—— (1955). Intracellular potentials recorded from a mammalian sympathetic ganglion. *J. Physiol.,* **130**: 572–84. [7, 13, 85, 87, 200]

—— (1956). Unpublished observations. [85, 87, 98, 183, 184, 205]

Edds, M. V. (1950). Hypertrophy of nerve fibres to functionally overloaded muscles. *J. comp. Neurol.,* **93**: 259–75. [236]

Eldred, E.; Granit, R.; and Merton, P. A. (1953). Supraspinal control of the muscle spindles and its significance. *J. Physiol.,* **122**: 498–523 [231]

——, and Hagbarth, K. E. (1954). Facilitation and inhibition of gamma efferents by stimulation of certain skin areas. *J. Neurophysiol.,* **17:** 59–65. [231]

Emmelin, N. G., and MacIntosh, F. C. (1948). Some conditions affecting the release of acetylcholine in sympathetic ganglia and skeletal muscles. *Acta physiol. scand., Suppl.,* **53:** 17–18. [198]

——, —— (1956). The release of acetylcholine from perfused sympathetic ganglia and skeletal muscles. *J. Physiol.,* **131:** 477–96. [182, 183, 198, 216]

——, and Muren, A. (1950). Acetylcholine release at parasympathetic synapses. *Acta physiol. scand.,* **20:** 13–32. [182]

Eyzaguirre, C., and Kuffler, S. W. (1955a). Processes of excitation in the dendrites and in the soma of single isolated sensory nerve cells of the lobster and crayfish. *J. Gen. Physiol.,* **39:** 87–119. [6, 7, 8, 13, 88, 89, 151]

——, —— (1955b). Further study of soma, dendrites and axon excitation in single neurons. *J. Gen. Physiol.,* **39:** 121–53. [8, 21, 53, 88, 90, 151, 225]

Fatt, P. (1954). Biophysics of junctional transmission. *Physiol. Rev.,* **34:** 674–710. [39, 132, 180, 182, 195, 215]

—— (1956a). Electric potentials around an antidromically activated motoneurone. *J. Neurophysiol.* In press. [50, 51, 227]

—— (1956b). Mode of activation of the motoneurone. *J. Neurophysiol.* In press. [40, 46, 49, 50]

——, and Katz, B. (1951). An analysis of the end-plate potential recorded with an intra-cellular electrode. *J. Physiol.,* **115:** 320–70. [5, 22, 35, 46, 52, 58, 181, 218, 220]

——, —— (1952). Spontaneous subthreshold activity at motor nerve endings. *J. Physiol.,* **117:** 109–128. [201, 203]

——, —— (1953). The effect of inhibitory nerve impulses on a crustacean muscle fibre. *J. Physiol.,* **121:** 374–89. [22, 98, 118, 128, 132, 133, 152]

Feldberg, W. (1945). Present views on the mode of action of acetylcholine in the central nervous system. *Physiol. Rev.,* **25:** 596–642. [182, 186]

—— (1950a). The role of acetylcholine in the central nervous system. *Brit. med. Bull.,* **6:** 312–21. [182]

—— (1950b). Gegenwärtige Probleme auf dem Gebeit der chemischen Übertragung von Nervenwirkungen. *Arch. exp. Path. Pharmak.,* **212:** 64–88. [182]

—— (1954). Central and sensory transmission. *Pharmacol. Rev.,* **6:** 85–93. [186, 191, 232]

——; Gray, J. A. B.; and Perry, W. L. M. (1953). Effects of close arterial injections of acetylcholine on the activity of the cervical spinal cord of the cat. *J. Physiol.,* **119:** 428–38. [186]

——, and Sherwood, S. L. (1954). Injections of drugs into the lateral ventricle of the cat. *J. Physiol.,* **123:** 148–67. [192]

——, and Vartiainen, A. (1934). Further observations on the physiology and pharmacology of a sympathetic ganglion. *J. Physiol.,* **83:** 103–28. [198]

——, and Vogt, M. (1948). Acetylcholine synthesis in different regions of the central nervous system. *J. Physiol.,* **107:** 372–81. [186, 187, 232]

Feng, T. P. (1941). Studies on the neuromuscular junction. XXVI. The changes of the end-plate potential during and after prolonged stimulation.

Chinese J. Physiol., 16: 341–72. [206, 207]

Fessard, A. (1946). Some basic aspects of the activity of electric plates. *Ann. N. Y. Acad. Sci.,* 47: 501–14. [52, 222]

—— (1952). Diversity of transmission processes as exemplified by specific synapses in electric organs. *Proc. Roy. Soc.,* B, 140: 186–91. [52, 222]

——, and Posternak, J. (1950). Les mecanismes elementaires de la transmission synaptique. *J. Physiologie,* 42: 319–437. [39, 52, 180, 182, 222]

Florey, Elizabeth, and Florey, E. (1955). Microanatomy of the abdominal stretch receptors of the crayfish *(Astacus fluviatilis 1.). J. Gen. Physiol.,* 39: 69–85. [7, 128]

Florey, E. (1954). An inhibitory and an excitatory factor of mammalian central nervous system, and their action on a single sensory neuron. *Arch. int. Physiol.,* 62: 33–53. [191]

——, and McLennan, H. (1955a). The release of an inhibitory substance from mammalian brain, and its effect on peripheral synaptic transmission. *J. Physiol.,* 129: 384–92. [197]

——, —— (1955b). Effects of an inhibitory factor (Factor I) from brain on central synaptic transmission. *J. Physiol.,* 130: 446–55. [197]

Forbes, A. (1934). The mechanism of reaction. In: *A Handbook of General Experimental Psychology.* Worcester, Clark Univ. Press. [55]

—— (1939). Problems of synaptic function. *J. Neurophysiol.,* 2: 465–72. [55]

Francis, C. M. (1953). Cholinesterase in the retina. *J. Physiol.,* 120: 435–39. [232]

Frank, K., and Fuortes, M. G. F. (1955a). Pre-spike potentials in elements of spinal cord. *Amer. J. Physiol.,* 183: 616–7. [8, 30]

——, —— (1955b). Potentials recorded from the spinal cord with microelectrodes. *J. Physiol.,* 130: 625–54. [8, 12, 30, 48, 69, 76, 84]

——, —— (1956a). Unitary activity of spinal interneurones of cats. *J. Physiol.,* 131: 424–35. [8, 84]

——, —— (1956b). Personal communication. [8, 16, 19, 40, 41, 50, 53]

Fuortes, M. G. F. (1954). Direct current stimulation of motoneurones. *J. Physiol.,* 126: 494–506. [66, 68]

Galambos, R. (1952). Microelectrode studies on medial geniculate body of cat. III. Response to pure tones. *J. Neurophysiol.,* 15: 381–400. [229]

——; Rose, J. E.; Bromiley, R. B.; and Hughes, J. H. (1952). Microelectrode studies on medial geniculate body of cat. II. Response to clicks. *J. Neurophysiology,* 15: 359–80. [229]

Gasser, H. S. (1939). Axons as samples of nervous tissue. *J. Neurophysiol.,* 2: 361–69. [82]

Gernandt, B. E., and Terzuolo, C. A. (1955). Effect of vestibular stimulation on strychnine-induced activity of the spinal cord. *Amer. J. Physiol.,* 183: 1–8. [198]

Gesell, R. (1940). A neurophysiological interpretation of the respiratory act. *Ergebn. Physiol.,* 43: 477–639. [55]

Glees, P., and Soler, J. (1951). Fibre content of the posterior column and synaptic connections of nucleus gracilis. *Z. Zellforsch.,* 36: 381–400. [176]

Goldman, D. E. (1943). Potential, impedance and rectification in membranes. *J. gen. Physiol.,* 27: 37–60. [123]

Granit, R. (1950). Reflex self-regulation of muscle contraction and autogenetic inhibition. *J. Neurophysiol.,* **13**: 351–72. [99]

────── (1955). *Receptors and Sensory Perception.* New Haven, Yale University Press. [178, 179, 231]

────── (1956). Reflex rebound by post-tetanic potentiation. Temporal summation—spasticity. *J. Physiol.,* **131**: 32–51. [210]

──────, and Kaada, B. R. (1952). Influence of stimulation of central nervous structures on muscle spindles in cat. *Acta physiol. scand.,* **27**: 130–60. [179, 231]

──────; Skoglund, S.; and Thesleff, S. (1953). Activation of muscle spindles by succinylcholine and decamethonium. The effects of curare. *Acta physiol. scand.,* **28**: 134–51. [189]

──────, and Ström, G. (1951). Autogenetic modulation of excitability of single ventral horn cells. *J. Neurophysiol.,* **14**: 113–32. [99]

Grundfest, H. (1955). Instrument requirements and specifications in bioelectric recording. *Ann. N. Y. Acad. Sci.,* **60**: 841–59. [8, 9]

──────, and Campbell, B. (1942). Origin, conduction and termination of impulses in the dorsal spino-cerebellar tract of cats. *J. Neurophysiol.,* **5**: 275–94. [175, 176]

──────, and Carter, W. B. (1954). Afferent relations of inferior olivary nucleus. 1. Electrophysiological demonstration of dorsal spino-olivary tract in cat. *J. Neurophysiol.,* **17**: 72–91. [231]

──────; Kao, C. Y.; and Altamirano, M. (1954). Bioelectric effects of ions injected into the giant axon of Loligo. *J. gen. Physiol.,* **38**: 245–82. [28]

Hagbarth, K. E. (1952). Excitatory and inhibitory skin areas for flexor and extensor motoneurones. *Acta physiol. scand.,* **26**: Suppl., 94. [99]

Haggar, R. A., and Barr, M. L. (1950). Quantitative data on the size of synaptic end-bulbs in the cat's spinal cord. *J. comp. Neurol.,* **93**: 17–35. [2]

van Harreveld, A. (1946). Asphyxial depolarisation in the spinal cord. *Amer. J. Physiol.,* **147**: 669–84. [27]

──────, and Feigen, G. A. (1948). Effect of nicotine on spinal synaptic conduction and on polarization of spinal cord. *J. Neurophysiol.,* **11**: 141–48. [184]

Harvey, A. M., and MacIntosh, F. C. (1940). Calcium and synaptic transmission in a sympathetic ganglion. *J. Physiol.,* **97**: 408–16. [204]

Hebb, C. O.; Silver, A.; Swan, A. A. B.; and Walsh, E. G. (1953). A histochemical study of cholinesterases of rabbit retina and optic nerve. *Quart. J. exp. Physiol.,* **38**: 185–91. [232]

Hellauer, H. F. (1953). Zur Charakterisierung der Erregungssubstanz sensiblen Nerven. *Arch. exp. Path. Pharmak.,* **219**: 234–41. [190]

──────, and Umrath, K. (1948). Uber die aktionssubstanz der sensiblen Nerven. *Pflüg. Arch. ges. Physiol.,* **249**: 619–30. [188, 190]

Hennemann, E.; Kaplan, A.; and Unna, K. (1949). A neuropharmacological study of the effect of myanesin (tolserol) on motor systems. *J. Pharmacol. exp. Therap.,* **97**: 331–41. [187]

Hess, A. (1953). The ground substance of the central nervous system revealed by histochemical staining. *J. comp. Neurol.,* **98**: 69–91. [217]

────── (1955). The ground substance of the developing central nervous system. *J. comp. Neurol.,* **102**: 65–75. [217]

van Heyningen, W. E. (1950). *Bacterial Toxins.* Oxford, Blackwell Scientific Publications. [196]

Hodgkin, A. L. (1947). The effect of potassium on the surface membrane of an isolated axon. *J. Physiol.,* **106:** 319–40. [221]

—— (1948). The local electric changes associated with repetitive action in a non-medullated axon. *J. Physiol.,* **107:** 165–81. [45, 65]

—— (1951). The ionic basis of electrical activity in nerve and muscle. *Biol. Rev.,* **26:** 339–409. [18, 22, 24, 71, 75, 92, 118, 126, 221]

——, and Huxley, A. F. (1952a). Currents carried by sodium and potassium ions through the membrane of the giant axon of *Loligo. J. Physiol.,* **116:** 449–72. [17]

——, —— (1952b). The components of membrane conductance in the giant axon of *Loligo. J. Physiol.,* **116:** 473–96. [17, 29, 126, 221]

——, —— (1952c). A quantitative description of membrane current and its application to conduction and excitation in nerve. *J. Physiol.,* **117:** 500–44. [38, 65, 71, 75, 221, 222]

——; ——; and Katz, B. (1952). Measurement of current-voltage relations in the membrane of the giant axon of *Loligo. J. Physiol.,* **116:** 424–48. [15, 17, 23, 38, 45, 77]

——, and Katz, B. (1949). The effect of sodium ions on the electrical activity of the giant axon of the squid. *J. Physiol.,* **108:** 37–77. [71, 123, 126]

——, and Keynes, R. D. (1953). The mobility and diffusion coefficient of potassium in giant axons from *Sepia. J. Physiol.,* **119:** 513–28. [23, 122]

——, —— (1955). Active transport of cations in giant axons from *Sepia* and *Loligo. J. Physiol.,* **128:** 28–60. [27, 28, 79, 82, 127]

Hoff, E. C. (1932a). Central nerve terminals in the mammalian spinal cord and their examination by experimental degeneration. *Proc. Roy. Soc.,* B, **111:** 175–88. [4, 52]

—— (1932b). The distribution of the spinal terminals (boutons) of the pyramidal tract, determined by experimental degeneration. *Proc. Roy. Soc.,* B, **111:** 226–37 [178]

—— (1935). Corticospinal fibers arising in the premotor area of the monkey. *Arch. Neurol. Psychiat., Chicago,* **33:** 687–97. [178]

——, and Hoff, H. E. (1934). Spinal terminations of the projection fibres from the motor cortex of primates. *Brain,* **57:** 454–74. [178]

Hoffmann, P. (1922). *Untersuchungen über die Eigenreflexe (Sehnenreflexe) menschlicher Muskeln.* Berlin, Springer. [188]

Holton, F. A., and Holton, P. (1954). The capillary dilator substances in dry powders of spinal roots; a possible role of adenosine triphosphate in chemical transmission from nerve endings. *J. Physiol.,* **126:** 124–40. [190]

Horstmann, E. (1954). Über kernspezifische Synapsenformen im Mittelhirn von Knockenfischen. *Z. Zellforsch,* **40:** 139–50. [218]

Howland, B.; Lettvin, J. Y.; McCulloch, W. S.; Pitts, W.; and Wall, P. D. (1955). Reflex inhibition by dorsal root interaction. *J. Neurophysiol.,* **18:** 1–17. [148]

Hunt, C. C. (1951). The reflex activity of mammalian small-nerve fibres. *J. Physiol.,* **115:** 456–69. [231]

—— (1954). Relation of function to diameter in afferent fibres of muscle nerves. *J. gen. Physiol.,* **38:** 117–31. [179]

—— (1955). Monosynaptic reflex response of spinal motoneurones to graded afferent stimulation. *J. gen. Physiol.,* **38:** 813–52. [39, 64]

Hutter, O. F., and Kostial, K. (1954). Effect of magnesium and calcium ions on the release of acetylcholine. *J. Physiol.,* **124:** 234–41. [204]

——, —— (1955). The relationship of sodium ions to the release of acetylcholine. *J. Physiol.,* **129:** 159–66. [204, 205]

——, and Trautwein, W. (1955). Vagal effects on the sinus venosus of the frog's heart. *J. Physiol.,* **129:** 48P. [98, 152]

Huxley, A. F. (1954). Electrical processes in nerve conduction. In: *Ion Transport Across Membranes,* 23–34. New York, Academic Press Inc. [221]

——, and Stampfli, R. (1949). Evidence for saltatory conduction in peripheral myelinated nerve fibres. *J. Physiol.,* **108:** 315–39. [181]

Hydén, H. (1943). Protein metabolism in the nerve cell during growth and function. *Acta physiol. scand.,* **6:** Suppl., 17. [5, 234]

Jefferson, A. A., and Benson, A. (1953). Some effects of post-tetanic potentiation of monosynaptic response of spinal cord of cat. *J. Neurophysiol.,* **16:** 381–96. [206]

——, and Schlapp, W. (1953). Some effects of repetitive stimulation of afferents on reflex conduction: In: *The Spinal Cord,* 99–119. Ciba Found. Symp. London, Churchill. [201]

Job, C., and Lundberg, A. (1953). On the significance of post- and presynaptic events for facilitation and inhibition in the sympathetic ganglion of the cat. *Acta physiol. scand.,* **28:** 14–28. [132, 206, 207]

Jung, R. (1953a). Allgemeine Neurophysiologie: Die Tätigkeit des Nerven systems. In: *Handbuch der inneren Medizin,* 1–181. Berlin, Göttingen, Heidelberg, Springer. [50, 162, 224, 225, 232, 233]

—— (1953b). Neuronal discharge. Symposia, Third Internat. EEG Congress 1953, 57–71. [85, 225]

——; v. Baumgarten, R.; and Baumgartner, G. (1952). Mikroableitungen von einzelnen Nervenzellen im optischen Cortex der Katze: Die licktaktivierten B-Neurone. *Arch. Psychiatr. und Zeits. Neurol.,* **189:** 521–39. [229]

——, and Baumgartner, G. (1955). Hemmungsmechanismen und bremsende Stabilisierung an einzelnen Neuron des optischen Cortex. *Pflüg. Arch. ges. Physiol.,* **261:** 434–56. [229]

Kaada, B. R. (1950). Site of action of myanesin (mephenesin, tolserol) in the central nervous system. *J. Neurophysiol.,* **13:** 89–108. [187, 188]

Kahlson, G., and MacIntosh, F. C. (1939). Acetylcholine synthesis in a sympathetic ganglion. *J. Physiol.,* **96:** 277–92. [198]

Kapera, H., and Lazarini, W. (1953). Zur frage der zentralen Ubertragung afferenter Impulse. IV. Die Verteilung der Substanz P im Zentralnervensystem. *Arch. exp. Path. Pharmak.,* **219:** 214–22. [191]

Katz, B. (1948). The electrical properties of the muscle fibre membrane. *Proc. Roy. Soc.,* B, **135:** 506–34. [18]

Keynes, R. D. (1954). The ionic fluxes in frog muscle. *Proc. Roy. Soc.,* B, **142:** 359–82. [29]

——, and Lewis, P. R. (1951). The sodium and potassium content of cephalopod nerve fibres. *J. Physiol.,* **114:** 151–82. [24]

Kirsche, W. (1950). Die regenerativen Vorgänge am Rückenmark erwachsener Teleostier nach operativer Kontinuitätstrennung. *Z. Mikr.-anat. Forsch.,* **56:** 190–265. [238]

Koechlin, B. A. (1954). The isolation and identification of the major anion fraction of the axoplasm of squid giant nerve fibres. *Proc. nat. Acad. Sci. Wash.*, **40**: 60–62. [27]

Koelle, G. B. (1954). The histochemical localization of cholinesterases in the central nervous system of the rat. *J. comp. Neurol.*, **100**: 211–35. [183, 187]

Krnjevic, K. (1955). The distribution of Na and K in cat nerves. *J. Physiol.*, **128**: 473–88. [24]

Kuffler, S. W. (1942). Further study on transmission in an isolated nerve-muscle fibre preparation. *J. Neurophysiol.*, **5**: 309–22. [35]

—— (1943). Specific excitability of the endplate region in normal and denervated muscle. *J. Neurophysiol.*, **6**: 99–110. [5]

—— (1944). The effect of calcium on the neuro-muscular junction. *J. Neurophysiol.*, **7**: 17–26. [203]

——, and Eyzaguirre, C. (1955). Synaptic inhibition in an isolated nerve cell. *J. Gen. Physiol.*, **39**: 155–84. [21, 98, 109, 128, 129, 130, 131, 149, 150]

——, and Vaughan Williams, E. M. (1953). Small-nerve junctional potentials. The distribution of small motor nerves to frog skeletal muscle, and the membrane characteristics of the fibres they innervate. *J. Physiol.*, **121**: 289–317. [52, 222]

Landolt-Börnstein, H. H. (1936). *Physikalisch-chemische Tabellen*, 5th ed., Book III, Part 3. Berlin, Springer. [116]

Laporte, Y., and Lloyd, D. P. C. (1952). Nature and significance of the reflex connections established by large afferent fibres of muscular origin. *Amer. J. Physiol.*, **169**: 609–21. [99, 134, 143, 144, 154, 157, 170, 171, 173]

——, and Lorente de Nó, R. (1950). Potential changes evoked in a curarized sympathetic ganglion by presynaptic volleys of impulses. *J. cell. comp. Physiol.*, **35**: Suppl. 2, 61–106. [98, 131, 183]

——; Lundberg, A.; and Oscarsson, O. (1956). Functional organization of the dorsal spino-cerebellar tract in the cat. II. Single fibre recording in the Fleschig's fasciculus on electrical stimulation of various peripheral nerves. *Acta physiol. scand.*, **36**: 188–203. [174, 176, 214, 229]

Larrabee, M. G., and Bronk, D. W. (1947). Prolonged facilitation of synaptic excitation in sympathetic ganglia. *J. Neurophysiol.*, **10**: 139–54. [200, 206, 207, 209]

Lembeck, F. (1953). Zur Frage der zentralen Ubertragung afferenter Impulse. *Arch. exp. Path. Pharmak.*, **219**: 197–213. [190, 191]

Lewis, P. R. (1952). The free amino-acids of invertebrate nerve. *Biochem. J.*, **52**: 330–38. [27]

Li, C. L., and Jasper, H. (1953). Microelectrode studies of the electrical activity of the cerebral cortex in the cat. *J. Physiol.*, **121**: 117–40. [85, 225]

Liley, A. W. (1956a). An investigation of spontaneous activity at the neuromuscular junction of the rat. *J. Physiol.*, **132**: 650–66. [209, 210, 211]

—— (1956b). The quantal components of the mammalian end-plate potential. *J. Physiol.*, **133**: 571–87. [202, 203]

—— (1956c). The effects of presynaptic polarization on the spontaneous activity of the mammalian neuro-muscular junction. *J. Physiol.* In press. [202]

——, and North, K. A. K. (1953). An electrical investigation of effects of repetitive stimulation on mammalian neuromuscular junction. *J. Neurophysiol.*, 16: 509–27. [200, 206, 208, 210, 211]

Lloyd, D. P. C. (1941a). Activity in neurons of the bulbospinal correlation system. *J. Neurophysiol.*, 4: 115–34. [179, 228]

——— (1941b). A direct central inhibitory action of dromically conducted impulses. *J. Neurophysiol.*, 4: 184–90. [97, 154]

——— (1941c). The spinal mechanism of the pyramidal system in cats. *J. Neurophysiol.*, 1941, 4: 525–46. [178, 179, 228]

——— (1942). Mediation of descending long spinal reflex activity. *J. Neurophysiol.*, 5: 435–58. [179, 228]

——— (1944). Functional organization of the spinal cord. *Physiol. Rev.*, 24: 1–17. [178, 180]

——— (1946). Facilitation and inhibition of spinal motoneurones. *J. Neurophysiol.*, 9: 421–38. [67, 97, 134, 143, 144, 154, 157]

——— (1949). Post-tetanic potentiation of response in monosynaptic reflex pathways of the spinal cord. *J. gen. Physiol.*, 33: 147–70. [206, 208, 210]

——— (1951a). Electrical signs of impulse conduction in spinal motoneurones. *J. gen. Physiol.*, 35: 255–88. [5, 49]

——— (1951b). After-currents, after-potentials, excitability, and ventral root electrotonus in spinal motoneurones. *J. gen. Physiol.*, 35: 289–321. [82, 83]

——— (1952a). Electrical manifestations of action in neurones. In: *The Biology of Mental Health and Disease,* 135–61. New York, Paul B. Hoeber. [36, 210]

——— (1952b). Electrotonus in dorsal nerve roots. *Cold Spr. Harb. Symp. quant. Biol.*, 17: 203–19. [206, 208]

——— (1953). Influence of asphyxia upon the responses of spinal motoneurones. *J. gen. Physiol.*, 36: 673–702. [27]

——— (1955). Synaptic transmission. In: *Textbook of Physiology,* edited by J. F. Fulton, 17th Edit. Philadelphia and London, W. B. Saunders. [36]

——— (1956). Monosynaptic reflex response as a function of frequency. Abstr. *XX Int. Physiol. Congr.*, 579–80. [68, 201]

———, and McIntyre, A. K. (1948). Analysis of forelimb-hindlimb reflex activity in acutely decapitate cats. *J. Neurophysiol.*, 11: 455–70. [228]

———, ——— (1949). On the origins of dorsal root potentials. *J. gen. Physiol.*, 32: 409–43. [36]

———, ——— (1950). Dorsal column conduction of group I muscle afferent impulses and their relay through Clarke's column. *J. Neurophysiol.*, 13: 39–54. [175]

———, ——— (1955). Monosynaptic reflex responses of individual motoneurones. *J. gen. Physiol.*, 38: 771–87. [39, 64]

Lorente de Nó, R. (1934). Studies on the structure of the cerebral cortex. II. Continuation of the study of the Ammonic system. *J. Psychol. Neurol. Lpz.*, 46: 113–77. [223]

——— (1938). Synaptic stimulation of motoneurones as a local process. *J. Neurophysiol.*, 1: 195–206. [4, 52, 55, 219, 223]

——— (1947). Action potential of the motoneurons of the hypoglossus nucleus. *J. cell. comp. Physiol.*, 29: 207–88. [49]

——— (1949). On the effect of certain quaternary ammonium ions upon frog nerve. *J. cell. comp. Physiol.*, 33: Suppl., 1–231. [221]

——— (1953). Conduction of impulses in the neurons of the oculomotor nucleus. In: *The Spinal Cord*, 132–173. Ciba Found. Symp. London, Churchill. [5, 49, 50, 227]

———, and Laporte, Y. (1950). Refractoriness, facilitation and inhibition in a sympathetic ganglion. *J. cell. comp. Physiol.*, 35: Suppl. 2, 155–92. [98, 132]

Lundberg, A. (1952). Adrenaline and transmission in the sympathetic ganglion of the cat. *Acta physiol. scand.*, 26: 252–63. [132]

McCouch, G. P.; Austin, G. M.; and Liu, C. Y. (1955). Sprouting of new terminals as a cause of spasticity. *Amer. J. Physiol.*, 183: 642–3. [237]

MacIntosh, F. C. (1938). Liberation of acetylcholine by the perfused superior cervical ganglion. *J. Physiol.*, 94: 155–69. [198]

——— (1941). The distribution of acetylcholine in the peripheral and central nervous system. *J. Physiol.*, 99: 436–42. [186]

———, and Oborin, P. E. (1953). Release of acetylcholine from intact cerebral cortex. XIX Internat. Physiol. Cong., Montreal. Abstracts of Communications. [187]

McLennan, H. (1954). Acetylcholine metabolism of normal and axotomized ganglia. *J. Physiol.*, 124: 113–16. [234]

Magladery, J. W., and Teasdale, R. D. (1956). Personal communication. [237]

Marrazzi, A. S. (1939). Adrenergic inhibition at sympathetic synapses. *Amer. J. Physiol.*, 127: 738–44. [132]

——— (1953). Some indications of cerebral humoral mechanisms. *Science*, 118: 367–70. [187, 192]

———, and Hart, E. R. (1955). Relationship of hallucinogens to adrenergic cerebral neurohumors. *Science*, 121: 365–67. [192]

Minz, B. (1955). *The role of humoral agents in nervous activity*. Springfield, Ill., Charles C. Thomas. [182]

Naess, K. (1950). The effect of D-tubocurarine on the mono- and polysynaptic reflex of the spinal cord including a comparison with the effect of strychnine. *Acta physiol. scand.*, 21: 34–40. [188]

Nastuk, W. L., and Hodgkin, A. L. (1950). The electrical activity of single muscle fibres. *J. cell. comp. Physiol.*, 35: 39–74. [58]

Niemer, W. T., and Magoun, H. W. (1947). Reticulo-spinal tracts influencing motor activity. *J. comp. Neurol.*, 87: 367–79. [228]

Ogston, A. G. (1955). Removal of acetylcholine from a limited volume by diffusion. *J. Physiol.*, 128: 222–23. [215]

Palade, G. E., and Palay, S. L. (1954). Electron microscope observations of interneuronal and neuromuscular synapses. *Anat. Rec.*, 118: 335–36. [4, 204, 205]

———, ——— (1956). Personal communication. [204, 205]

Palay, S. L., and Palade, G. E. (1955). The fine structure of neurons. *J. Biophys. Biochem. Cytology*, 1: 69–88. [5, 234]

Parrot, J. L. (1954). The place of histamine in neurohumoral transmission. *Pharmacol. Rev.*, 6: 119–22. [192]

Patek, P. R. (1944). The perivascular spaces of the mammalian brain. *Anat. Rec.*, 88: 1–24. [189]

Perl, E. R., and Whitlock, D. G. (1955). Potentials evoked in cerebral somatosensory region. *J. Neurophysiol.*, **18**: 486–501. [225]

Pernow, B. (1953). Studies on substance P. Purification, occurrence and biological actions. *Acta physiol. scand.*, **29**: Suppl., 105. [190]

Perry, W. L. M. (1953). Acetylcholine release in the cat's superior cervical ganglion. *J. Physiol.*, **119**: 439–54. [183, 198, 199, 200]

——, and Talesnik, J. (1953). The role of acetylcholine in synaptic transmission at parasympathetic ganglia. *J. Physiol.*, **119**: 455–69. [182, 232]

Phillips, C. G. (1955). The dimensions of a cortical motor point. *J. Physiol.*, **129**: 20–21P. [8, 12, 85]

—— (1956a). Intracellular records from Betz cells in the cat. *Quart. J. exp. Physiol.*, **41**: 58–69. [8, 12, 85, 86]

—— (1956b). Cortical motor threshold and the thresholds and distribution of excited Betz cells in the cat. *Quart. J. exp. Physiol.*, **41**: 70–84. [8, 12, 41, 85, 86]

Renshaw, B. (1941). Influence of discharge of motoneurons upon excitation of neighbouring motoneurons. *J. Neurophysiol.*, **4**: 167–83. [162, 167]

—— (1942). Reflex discharges in branches of crural nerve. *J. Neurophysiol.*, **5**: 487–98. [97, 99]

—— (1946a). Central effects of centripetal impulses in axons of spinal ventral roots. *J. Neurophysiol.*, **9**: 191–204. [162]

—— (1946b). Observations on interaction of nerve impulses in the gray matter and on the nature of central inhibition. *Amer. J. Physiol.*, **146**: 443–48. [36, 148]

——; Forbes, A.; and Morison, B. R. (1940). Activity of isocortex and hippocampus: electrical studies with microelectrodes. *J. Neurophysiol.*, **3**: 74–105. [223]

de Robertis, E. D. P., and Bennett, H. S. (1955). Some features of the submicroscopic morphology of synapses in frog and earthworm. *J. Biophys. Biochem. Cytol.*, **1**: 47–58. [4, 204, 205]

Robertson, J. D. (1956). The ultrastructure of a reptilian myoneural junction. *J. Biophys. Biochem. Cytol.* In press. [4, 204, 205]

Rodriguez, L. A. (1955). Experiments on the histologic locus of the hematoencephalic barrier. *J. comp. Neurol.*, **102**: 27–45. [189]

Romanes, G. J. (1953). The motor cell groupings of the spinal cord. In: *The Spinal Cord*, 24–38. Ciba Found. Symp. London, Churchill. [229]

Rose, J. E., and Mountcastle, V. B. (1954). Activity of single neurones in the tactile thalamic region of the cat in response to a transient peripheral stimulus. *Johns Hopk. Hosp. Bull.*, **94**: 238–82. [41, 229]

Schaefer, H., and Haass, P. (1939). Über einen lokalen Erregungsstrom an der motorischen Endplatte. *Pflüg. Arch. ges. Physiol.*, **242**: 364–81. [206]

Scheibel, M. E., and Scheibel, A. B. (1955). The inferior olive. A Golgi study. *J. comp. Neurol.*, **102**: 77–132. [230]

——; ——; Mollica, A.; and Moruzzi, G. (1955). Convergence and interaction of afferent impulses on single units of reticular formation. *J. Neurophysiol.*, **18**: 309–31. [229]

Scherrer, J. (1952). Action de strychnine sur l'activite spinale reflexe. *J. Physiol. Path. gen.*, **44**: 29–44. [188]

Schimert, J. (1938). Die Endigungsweise des Tractus vestibulospiralis. *Z. Anat. Entw-Gesch.*, **108**: 761–67. [179]

—— (1939). Das Verhalten der Hinterwurzelkollateralen im Rücken-mark. *Z. Anat. Entw-Gesch.,* **109:** 665–87. [153, 158]

Schweitzer, A., and Wright, S. (1937a). The action of eserine and related compounds and of acetylcholine on the central nervous system. *J. Physiol.,* **89:** 165–97. [184]

——, —— (1937b). Further observations on the action of acetylcholine, prostigmine and related substances on the knee jerk. *J. Physiol.,* **89:** 384–402. [184]

——, —— (1938). Action of nicotine on the spinal cord. *J. Physiol.,* **94:** 136–47. [184]

Scott, D., and Clemente, C. D. (1955). Regeneration of spinal cord fibres in the cat. *J. comp. Neurol.,* **102:** 633–69. [237]

Shanes, A. M., and Berman, M. D. (1955). Kinetics of ion movement in the squid giant axon. *J. gen. Physiol.,* **39:** 279–300. [126, 127]

——; Grundfest, H.; and Freygang, W. (1953). Low level impedance changes following the spike in the squid giant axon before and after treatment with "veratrine" alkaloids. *J. gen. Physiol.,* **37:** 39–51. [126]

Sherrington, C. S. (1897). The central nervous system. In: Sir Michael Foster's *A Text Book of Physiology,* 7th Ed. London, Macmillan and Co. [1]

—— (1906). *The Integrative Action of the Nervous System.* New Haven and London, Yale University Press. [2, 195]

—— (1925). Remarks on some aspects of reflex inhibition. *Proc. Roy. Soc.,* B. **97:** 519–45. [2, 31, 100]

—— (1929). Some functional problems attaching to convergence. *Proc. Roy. Soc.,* B, **105:** 332–62. [2, 31]

—— (1931). Quantitative management of contraction in lowest level co-ordination. *Brain,* **54:** 1–28. [2]

Sholl, D. A. (1953). Dendritic organization in the neurons of the visual and motor cortices of the cat. *J. Anat.,* **87:** 387–406. [7, 225]

Skoglund, C. R. (1952). Factors that modify transmission through the spinal cord. *Cold Spr. Harb. Symp. quant. Biol.,* **17:** 233–44. [189]

Sperry, R. W. (1945). The problem of central nervous reorganization after nerve regeneration and muscle transposition. *Quart. Rev. Biol.,* **20:** 311–69. [237]

—— (1951). Mechanisms of neural maturation. In: *Handbook of Experimental Psychology,* edited by S. S. Stevens. New York, John Wiley and Sons. [238]

Sprague, J. M. (1956). Anatomical localisation of excitation and inhibition of spinal motoneurones. Abstr. XX Int. Physiol. Congr., 849–50. [156]

Ström, G. (1951). Physiological significance of post-tetanic potentiation of the spinal monosynaptic reflex. *Acta physiol. scand.,* **24:** 61–83. [206, 208, 209]

Szentágothai-Schimert, J. (1941). Die Endigungsweise der absteigenden Rückenmarksbahnen. *Z. Anat. Entw-Gesch.,* **111:** 322–30. [178, 179]

—— (1951). Short propriospinal neurons and intrinsic connections of the spinal gray matter. *Acta morphologica Hung.,* **1:** 81–94. [161, 178, 179, 228]

——, and Albert, A. (1955). The synaptology of Clarke's column. *Acta morphologica Hung.,* **5:** 43–51. [175, 176, 218]

———; Donhoffer, A.; and Rajkovits, K. (1955). Die Lokalisation der Cholinesterase in der interneuronalen Synapse. *Acta histochem.*, 1: 272–81. [215]

———, and Rajkovits, K. (1955). Die Rückwirkung der spezifischen Funktion auf die Struktur der Nervenelemente. *Acta morphol. Hung.*, 5: 253–74. [235, 236]

Taboada, R. P. (1927). Note sur la structure du corps genouillé externe. *Trab. Lab. Invest. biol. Univ. Madr.*, 25: 319–29. [230]

Tasaki, I. (1953). *Nervous Transmission.* Springfield, Ill., Charles C. Thomas. [181]

——— (1955). New measurements of the capacity and the resistance of the myelin sheath and the nodal membrane of the isolated frog nerve fibre. *Amer. J. Physiol.*, 181: 639–50. [181]

———; Hagiwara, S.; and Watanabe, A. (1954). Action potentials recorded from inside a Mauthner cell of the catfish. *Jap. J. Physiol.*, 4: 79–90. [224]

———; Polley, E. H.; and Orrego, F. (1954). Action potentials from individual elements in cat geniculate and striate cortex. *J. Neurophysiol.*, 17: 454–74. [41, 177, 229]

Tauc, L. (1954). Réponse de la cellule nerveuse du ganglion abdominal de *Aplysia depilans* à la stimulation directe intracellulaire. *C. R. Acad. Sci. Paris*, 339: 1537–39. [6, 7, 8, 13]

Tauc, L. (1955a). Réponse de la cellule nerveuse du ganglion abdominal d'*Aplysia punctata* activée par voie synaptique. *J. Physiologie*, 47: 286–87. [93]

——— (1955b). Étude de l'activité élémentaire des cellules du ganglion abdominal de l'Aplysie. *J. Physiologie*, 47: 769–92. [6, 7, 8, 13, 16, 20, 22, 93]

Taugner, R., and Culp, W. (1953). Über die Wirkung von Nicotin auf das Rückenmark der Katze. Einflüsse von Nicotin auf Patellarsehnen-, Flexor- und Extensor-reflex vor und nach Zufuhr von Interneuronengiften. *Arch. exper. Path. Pharmak.*, 220: 423–32. [184, 186]

Taverner, D. (1952). The action of alpha-beta-dihydroxy-gamma-(2-methylphenoxy)-propane (myanesin) on the spinal cord of the cat. *Brit. J. Pharmacol.*, 7: 655–64. [188]

Therman, P. O. (1941). Transmission of impulses through the Burdach nucleus. *J. Neurophysiol.*, 4: 153–66. [176]

Toennies, J. F., and Jung, R. (1948). Über rasch wiederholte Entladungen der Motoneurone und die Hemmungsphase des Beugereflexes. *Pflüg. Arch. ges. Physiol.*, 250: 667–93. [50]

Tschirgi, R. D. (1952). Blood-Brain Barrier, *The Biology of Mental Health and Disease,* 34–46. New York, Paul B. Hoeber, Inc. [189]

Umrath, K. (1953a). Der fermentative Abbau der Erregungssubstanz der sensiblen Nerven, seine pH-Abhängigkeit und seine Hemmung durch zentral erregende Stoffe. *Arch. exp. Path. Pharmak.*, 219: 148–55. [188, 190]

——— (1953b). Über die fermentative Verwandlung von substanz P aus sensiblen Neuronen in die Errungssubstanz der sensiblen Nerven. *Pflüg. Arch. ges. Physiol.*, 258: 230–42. [191]

Vogt, M. (1954). The concentration of sympathin in different parts of the central nervous system under normal conditions and after the administration of drugs. *J. Physiol.*, **123**: 451–81. [191, 192]

Weiss, P. (1952). Central versus peripheral factors in the development of coordination. *Res. Publ. Assn. nerv. ment. Dis.*, **30**: 3–23. [238]

Wiersma, C. A. G.; Furshpan, E.; and Florey, E. (1953). Physiological and pharmacological observations on muscle receptors of the crayfish, *Cambarus Clarkii* Girard. *J. exp. Biol.*, **30**: 136–50. [88]

Woodbury, J. W., and Patton, H. D. (1952). Electrical activity of single spinal cord elements. *Cold Spr. Harb. Symp. quant. Biol.*, **17**: 185–88. [7, 12, 30, 48, 69, 77]

Woollam, D. H. M., and Millen, J. W. (1954). Perivascular spaces of the mammalian central nervous system. *Biol. Rev.*, **29**: 251–83. [189]

Wright, E. B. (1954). Effect of Mephenesin and other "depressants" on spinal cord transmission in frog and cat. *Amer. J. Physiol.*, **179**: 390–401. [188]

Wyckoff, R. W. G., and Young, J. Z. (1956). The motoneurone surface. *Proc. Roy. Soc.*, B. **144**: 440–50. [3, 4, 51, 217, 223]

Young, J. Z. (1939). Fused neurones and synaptic contacts in the giant nerve fibres of cephalopods. *Phil. Trans. Roy. Soc.*, B, **229**: 465–503. [91, 92]

SYMBOLS

mm	= millimetre
μ	= 10^{-3} mm
Å	= Angstrom, 10^{-7} mm
p mole	= 10^{-12} moles
M	= mole per litre
m M	= 10^{-3} moles per litre
p equiv.	= 10^{-12} equivalents
msec.	= 10^{-3} seconds
μsec.	= 10^{-6} seconds
A	= Ampere
Ω	= ohm
M Ω	= 10^{6} ohms
V	= volt
mV	= 10^{-3} volt
μV	= 10^{-6} volt
F	= Farad
μF	= 10^{-6} Farad
$\mu\mu$F	= 10^{-12} Farad
mho	= reciprocal ohm

INDEX